Learn Clinical Reasoning in

Cardiology Through Cases

Learn Clinical Reasoning in

Cardiology Through Cases

Shyam S Kothari MD, DM
Professor of Cardiology (Retd.)
All India Institute of Medical Sciences
New Delhi, India

JAYPEE

JAYPEE BROTHERS MEDICAL PUBLISHERS
The Health Sciences Publisher
New Delhi | London

Jaypee Brothers Medical Publishers (P) Ltd

Headquarters
EMCA House, 23/23-B
Ansari Road, Daryaganj
New Delhi 110 002, India
Landline: +91-11-23272143, +91-11-23272703
+91-11-23282021, +91-11-23245672
e-mail: jaypee@jaypeebrothers.com

Corporate Office
4838/24, Ansari Road, Daryaganj
New Delhi 110 002, India
Phone: +91-11-43574357
Fax: +91-11-43574314
e-mail: jaypee@jaypeebrothers.com

Overseas Office
JP Medical Ltd.
83, Victoria Street, London
SW1H 0HW (UK)
Phone: +44-20 3170 8910
e-mail: info@jpmedpub.com

EU GPSR Authorised Representative
Logos Europe, 9 rue Nicolas Poussin
17000, La Rochelle, France
Phone: +33 (0) 6 67 93 73 78
e-mail: contact@logoseurope.eu

Website: www.jaypeebrothers.com
Website: www.jaypeedigital.com

Inquiries for bulk sales may be solicited at: jaypee@jaypeebrothers.com

Learn Clinical Reasoning in Cardiology Through Cases

First Edition: **2026**

ISBN: 978-93-6616-249-2

Printed at Officenow India

Dedicated to

the sense of wonderment in you.

Preface

Most probably, this book will not provide any new information to you. Equally likely, it would open some new windows for you to make a correct clinical diagnosis. The current crisis in clinical medicine does not stem from the lack of information but rather from the excess of information and lack of discriminatory intelligence which is not taught in contemporary cardiology courses. Instead, the students are encouraged to follow algorithms, checklists, and guidelines in order to deliver a standard of care. Unfortunately, the result is rote learning and numbing of discriminatory intelligence.

This small book just eclectically picks up a few cases that have been seen by the author and charts a course of enquiry through them to stimulate clinical thinking. The book does not claim to cover a significant portion of cardiology. In fact, it covers very little cardiology curriculum but attempts to uncover the patterns of thinking useful in making clinical diagnosis under all circumstances. It teaches rules by showing the exceptions. It should be useful to fellows in cardiology, pediatric cardiology, and internal medicine or anyone else who is a bit curious!

The best way to use this book is not to rush through the cases, but rather pause and try hard to seek your own answers before reading the "mundane" answers given in the book. That way you could learn more from yourself and teach the author as well.

You could potentially finish this small book over a weekend, but if you seriously ponder over the issues as envisaged in the book, it can be a transformative experience in clinical reasoning, even if a small one!

Happy reading.

Shyam S Kothari
(kothariss100@gmail.com)

Acknowledgments

The ideas and materials in this book are the result of my interaction with faculty colleagues and fellows at the All India Institute of Medical Sciences, New Delhi, India, for over 3 decades. I express my sincere thanks to all of them. More recently, the colleagues and students at the UN Mehta Institute of Cardiology, Ahmedabad, Gujarat have also added valuable stuff to the endeavor. Some of the videos or pictures have been provided by other colleagues that have been acknowledged at appropriate places.

I also thank the team at M/s Jaypee Brothers Medical Publishers (P) Ltd, New Delhi for accepting this unconventional book idea and doing a great job of it.

Finally, I thank the patients whose stories feature in this book that provide valuable lessons to us all, and also thank the students in anticipation, who would read this book and imbibe the lessons.

Contents

CASE

1

Prosthetic Heart Valve Thrombosis

"I cannot teach anybody anything. I can only make them think."

—Socrates

A 30-year-old man had mitral valve replacement with a mechanical prosthetic mitral valve for calcific rheumatic mitral stenosis. He suffered from two episodes of prosthetic heart valve thrombosis (PHVT). The PHVT episodes were treated with thrombolysis, but the second episode responded only partially. Subsequently, the mechanical valve was replaced with a bioprosthetic mitral valve. He was on regular follow-up. The last follow-up 6 months earlier showed well-functioning mitral bioprosthesis. He reported a recent increase in breathlessness for 1 month and the echo-Doppler is shown below (upper strip, **Figs. 1A and B, Videos 1 and 2**). The echo in **Figures 1C and D** and **Videos 3 and 4** were obtained after some treatment.

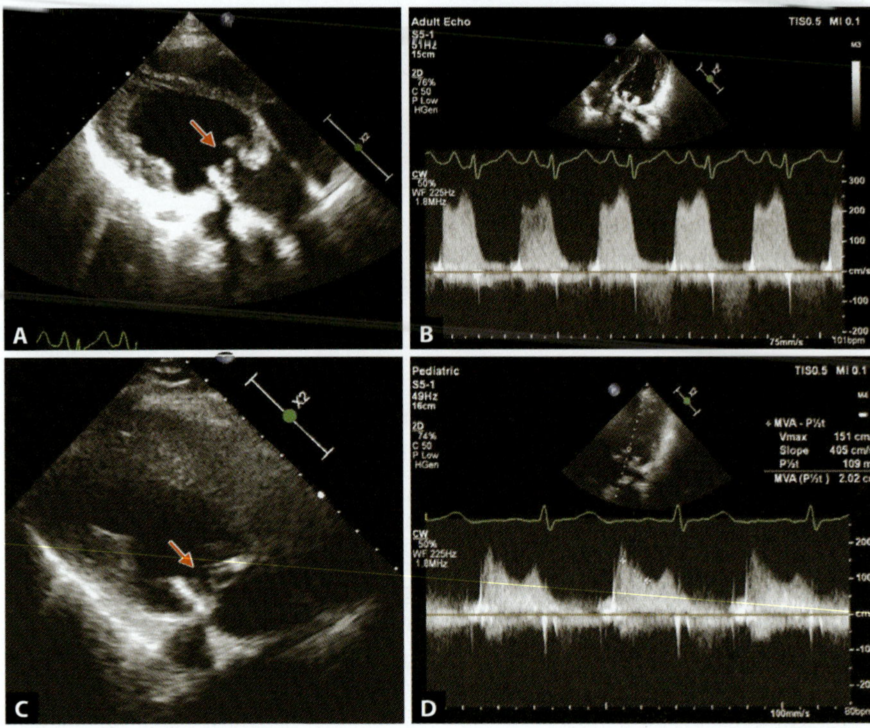

Figs. 1A to D: (A) Thickened and incompletely opening mitral valve bioprosthesis with high Doppler gradients (B) suggestive of prosthetic heart valve thrombosis (PHVT). (C and D) Thinned leaflets and markedly reduce gradients across mitral valve after treatment **(*see* Videos 1, 2, 3, and 4 also)**.

He was not thrombolyzed or reoperated. What could be the possible diagnosis and treatment?

Video 1 Video 2 Video 3 Video 4

Pause and think before you click the answer:

Answer: The patient suffered from bioprosthetic valve thrombosis as seen by the high gradients across mitral valve in Figure 1B. The change was recent and therefore it was not like a bioprosthetic valve degeneration. Further, it has improved. This patient had recurrent prosthetic valve thrombosis of mechanical valve previously and therefore a bioprosthesis was implanted. Unfortunately, the bioprosthesis also showed thrombosis.

The cause of PHVT in this patient was eosinophilia-induced thrombosis. On this admission, he had eosinophilia (77%) with an absolute eosinophilic count of 25,000/mm^3. The thrombosis disappeared after treatment with steroids, diethylcarbamazine, and heparin as seen in Figures 1C and D.

Learning points: Eosinophilia-induced thrombosis remains an under-recognized entity despite many case reports. Several cases of recurrent PHVT have been published where the eosinophilia has not been recognized and repeat surgeries have been performed for the PHVT, resulting in rethrombosis. Obviously, eosinophilia needs to be treated to prevent the recurrences. The treatment of eosinophilia would depend on the cause of eosinophilia. Eosinophilia-induced thrombosis might occur despite recommended international normalized ratio (INR). These patients may be maintained on a higher INR, but that is empirical. At least some cases of PHVT in Indian settings might be due to eosinophilia (that is not uncommonly seen in general population). Eosinophils cause thrombosis due to cationic protein release as seen in Loffler's syndrome resulting in ventricular thrombosis and endomyocardial fibrosis.

(*Source:* Kothari SS, Deepti S, Rai N. Reversible bioprosthetic valve thrombosis from eosinophilia. BMJ Case Rep. 2018 Feb 8;2018:bcr2017222937. doi: 10.1136/bcr-2017-222937.)

Sidelights:

1. **Can you have normal Doppler gradients with PHVT?**
2. **Which is a better test for PHVT-echocardiography or fluoroscopy?**
3. **Does thrombolytic therapy influence prothrombin time (PT) and activated partial thromboplastin time (aPTT)?**
4. **Why PHVT is more common in Indian patients?**
5. **What happens to patients with 1 leaflet of a bileaflet prosthetic heart valve partially stuck?**

(*Sidelights are food for thought—provided to increase your curiosity:* So as a rule, do not read these answers before you try to answer them yourself. The answers provided here are not intended to be exhaustive.)

Answer: The Doppler gradients may not be high if only 1 leaflet of a bileaflet prosthetic valve is stuck, or the valve area is not much compromised despite the thrombus, although absolutely normal gradients or a completely normal pattern would be uncommon. Because of this fact, fluoroscopic examination is preferred for PHVT if the prosthetic valve is seen on fluoroscopy (TTK chitra valve is not seen on fluoroscopy).

- Thrombolytic therapy prolongs both PT and aPTT.
- Most Indian series of patients with PHVT report a much higher incidence of PHVT in patients than that reported from the other parts of the world (6–10/100 patient years in India vs. 0.3–1.3/100 patient years in western series). PHVT is common in Indian patients due to several reasons. Less adequate INR monitoring, less time in therapeutic range, dietary variations, and poor patient compliance are the commonly cited reasons. However, an equally important reason also is that the patients are operated late with higher prevalence of large left atria, atrial fibrillation, and ventricular dysfunction amongst other factors.
- The fate of patient with 1 leaflet stuck after thrombolytic therapy for PHVT (when they are hemodynamically stable and symptomatically better) is not well known. Many patients are on follow-up with high INR due to unavailability/unfeasibility of repeat surgery; however, repeat PHVT with sudden deterioration might occur. It seems an unwise strategy to follow these patients on high INR only. Very careful follow-up is mandatory. Large objective data regarding this subset of patients are not available.

CASE

2

Dilated Cardiomyopathy

Life is short, the art long,
opportunity fleeting,
experiment uncertain,
and judgment difficult...

—Hippocrates

A 42-year-old woman presented to the emergency services in cardiogenic shock. She had a history of progressively worsening breathlessness for the past year; however, no medical evaluation had been done earlier. At presentation, her pulse was 110 beats/min, regular, and low volume, and the blood pressure was 90/70 mm Hg. On auscultation, third heart sound was present, but no murmurs were heard. Soon after presentation, she had an asystolic cardiac arrest. However, she was resuscitated successfully and mechanically ventilated. She required inotropic support with dopamine and noradrenaline for maintaining blood pressure. Her ECG showed normal sinus rhythm and nonspecific ST-T changes. Her chest X-ray is shown in **Figure 1A**. She had severe left ventricular (LV) dysfunction on echo with a LV ejection fraction (LVEF) of 20% **(Fig. 2A)**. She remained markedly symptomatic with fatigue and complained of blackouts on getting up. There was a postural drop of 25 mm Hg in systolic blood pressure on sitting up. Furthermore, it was noticed that her heart rates did not go beyond 110 beats/min, despite being on high doses of inotropes and remaining hypotensive. Patient's photograph is shown in **Figure 3**. Her chest X-ray and echo after 3 months are shown in **Figures 1B and 2B**.

Every physician would like to have such an outcome in his/her patients. But this was the result of physician's involvement with the patient, thoughtful observation and then asking past history!

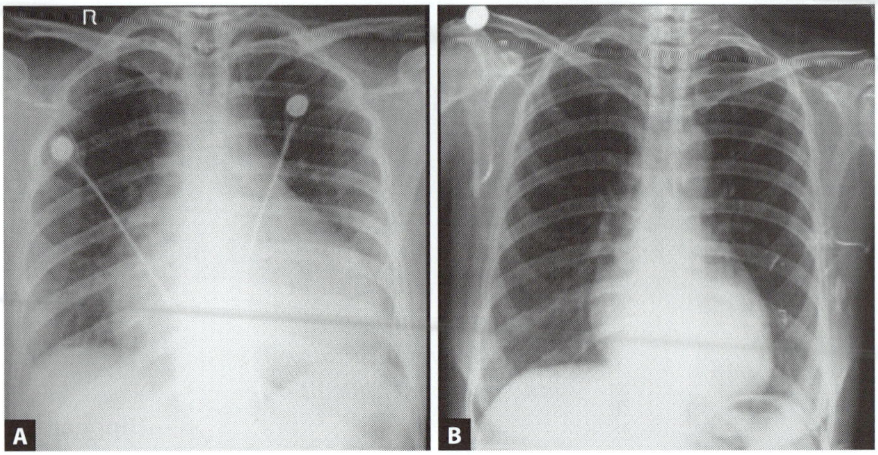

Figs. 1A and B: (A) Chest X-ray at admission; (B) After 6 months.

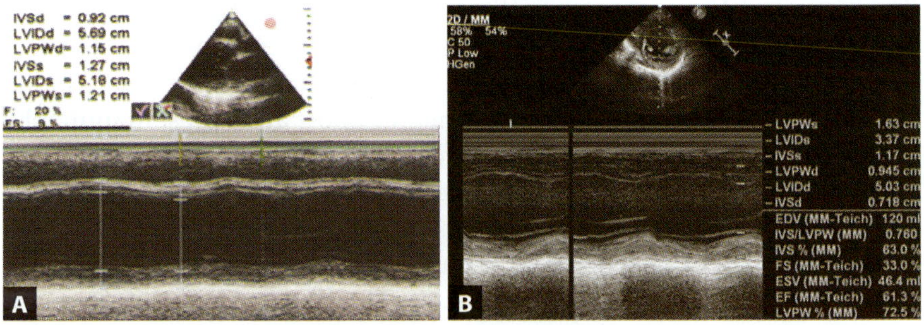

Figs. 2A and B: (A) M-mode echo at admission; (B) After 3 months.

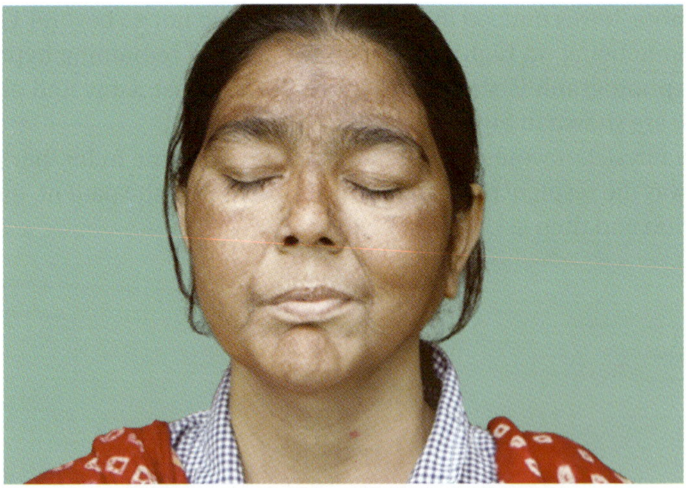

Fig. 3: Patient's photograph (with permission).

Can you guess the possible diagnosis?

Pause and think before you click the answer:

Answer: Her heart rate did not increase >110 beats/min despite inotropes and she would become dizzy on standing up. She had postural hypotension of 25 mm Hg. On close scrutiny, patchy pigmentation of face was noticed along with loss of axillary and pubic hair.

This observation arose suspicion of Addison's disease and a careful past history revealed that she had nearly bled to death in the last pregnancy 14 years earlier, and since then she did not have lactation or menstruation. The evaluation led to suspicion of Sheehan syndrome and the investigations confirmed it. She was treated with glucocorticoids, thyroxine, and fludrocortisone with remarkable results. She could be weaned off the inotropes in 2 days, and on follow-up 6 months later, the heart had recovered. Her pituitary hormones profile and the magnetic resonance imaging (MRI) showing cerebrospinal fluid (CSF)-filled empty sella are shown in the **Table 1** and **Figure 4**.

TABLE 1: Patient's hormone profile.

Hormone, unit	*Patient's value*	*Normal range*
Tri-iodothyronine, (T3), ng/mL	0.37	0.58–1.59
Thyroxine (T4), µg/dL	3.56	4.86–11.72
Thyroid-stimulating hormone, mIU/mL	1.92	0.35–4.94
Prolactin, ng/mL	<0.6	5.18–26.53
Follicle-stimulating hormone, mIU/mL	2.26	26.7–133.41
Luteinizing hormone, mIU/mL	0.76	10.39–64.75
Growth hormone, ng/mL	0.5	0.5–17
Fasting cortisol, µg/dL	6.0	5–25

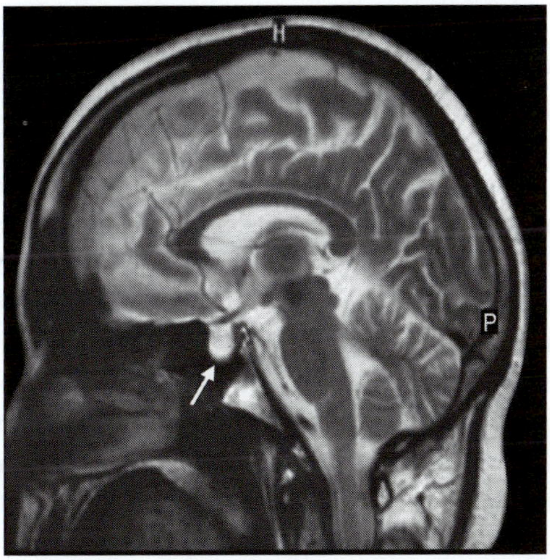

Fig. 4: MRI showing CSF-filled empty sella (arrow). (CSF: cerebrospinal fluid; MRI: magnetic resonance imaging)

(*Source:* Doshi S, Roy A, Ramamoorthy A, Kothari SS, Bahl VK. Dilated cardiomyopathy: a ghost from the past. Circ Heart Fail. 2013;6(2):e19-21.)

Learning points: Hypothyroidism, adrenal insufficiency, and growth hormone deficiency, individually, have been associated with heart failure, and with reversal of heart failure on hormone replacement. Thus, reversible heart failure attributable to collective deficiency of all these hormones, as in panhypopituitarism might occur, but rarely reported. This case highlights the importance of history, physical examination in the evaluation of patients, and adds Sheehan syndrome as a cause of reversible cardiomyopathy. But most of all, it is the ability of the physician to think contextually and investigate appropriately that is important, because every depigmented face is not Addison's disease, nor every postural hypotension!

Sidelights: Enumerate the causes of reversible LV systolic dysfunction?

(*Sidelights are food for thought—provided to increase your curiosity:* So as a rule, do not read these answers before you try to answer them yourself. The answers provided here are not intended to be exhaustive.)

Answer: Usual causes of reversible LV dysfunction include severe hypertension, aortic stenosis, coronary artery disease, thiamine deficiency, tachycardiomyopathy, endocrinopathies such as hypothyroidism and pheochromocytoma, metabolic causes such as hypoglycemia, hypocalcemia, and hypoxia, severe anemia, drugs and toxins, alcohol, infectious myocarditis, sarcoidosis, Takayasu aortoarteritis, Keshan disease, coronary vasculitis, severe obesity(!), Vit D deficiency(?), electrolyte disturbances, severe malnutrition, Takotsubo cardiomyopathy, chronic preload deprivation, etc.

It is important to realize that small changes in these reversible factors might be clinically meaningful for a patient with otherwise irreversible LV dysfunction such as dilated cardiomyopathy, and these things should be carefully sought and corrected in all patients with heart failure.

Coronary artery disease as a cause of reversible LV dysfunction needs to be carefully considered and is often misunderstood. Presence of coronary artery disease does not mean that it is a cause of LV dysfunction unless it is severe proximal disease causing significant ischemia at rest or repetitive ischemia on exertion. Only tight proximal severe multivessel disease will cause resting LV dysfunction. Thus, moderate triple vessel disease without a myocardial infarction will not cause LV dysfunction.

CASE

3

Ventricular Tachycardia

"To me the very essence of education is concentration of mind, not the collecting of facts. If I had to do my education over again, and had any voice in the matter, I would not study facts at all. I would develop the power of concentration and detachment, and then with a perfect instrument I could collect facts at will."

—Swami Vivekananda

A 59-year-old lady, was brought to emergency services in shock and altered sensorium. She had history of vomiting in the previous week, and had episodic unconsciousness four times in the last week. She received cardioversion at three different places for unconsciousness due to ventricular tachycardia (VT) prior to coming at this emergency **(Fig. 1)**. On examination, she had pulse of 56 beats/min, BP-80/60 mm Hg and altered sensorium. The oximetric saturation was 96%. The heart sounds were normal and bibasilar crepts were heard. Her ECG and X-rays are shown below **(Figs. 2 and 3)**. The echo showed mild left ventricular (LV) dysfunction, with LV ejection fraction (LVEF) of 35%, with no other abnormality.

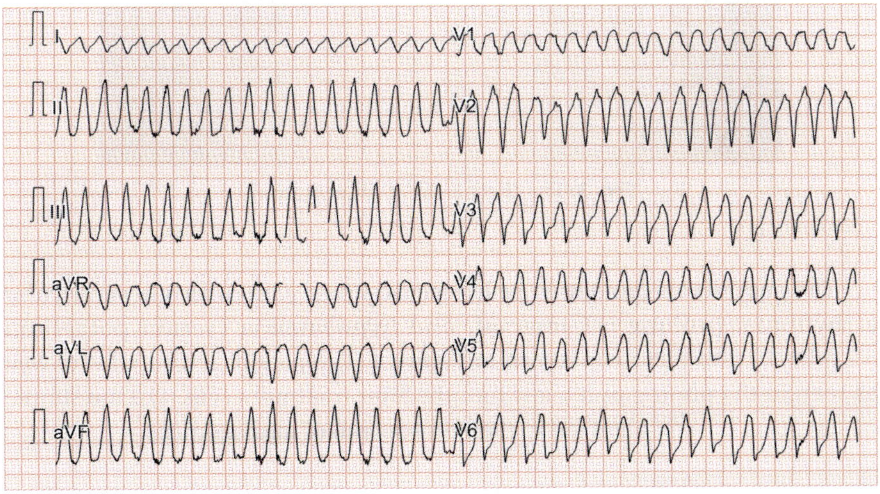

Fig. 1: ECG done in a prior hospital before cardioversion.

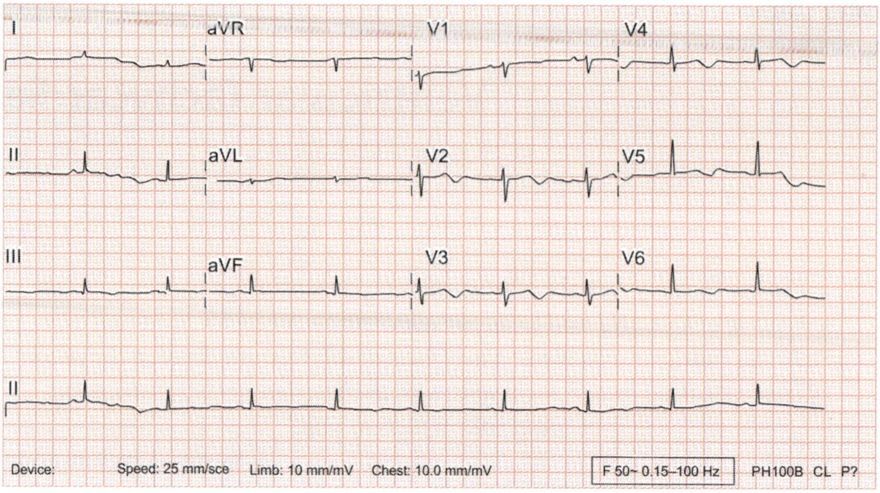

Fig. 2: The ECG at presentation to emergency.

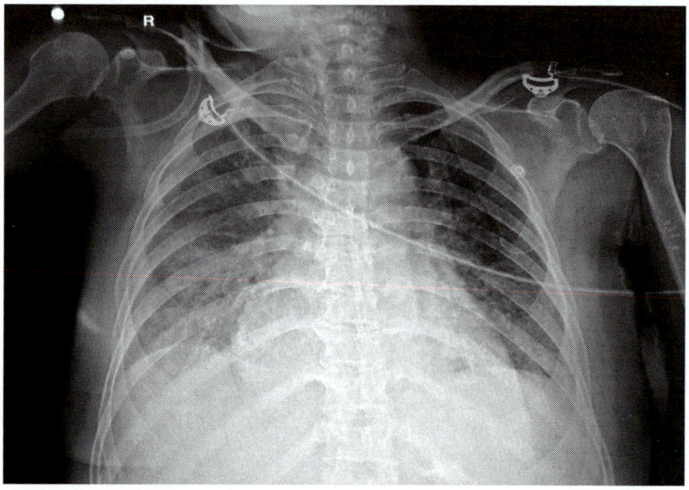

Fig. 3: The chest X-ray at presentation.

The patient was thought to be in electric storm with recurrent ventricular arrhythmia, prolong QT interval, and hypokalemia (serum potassium 3.2 mEq/L). Her picture is shown in **Figure 4**. The patient recovered very well as seen in the photograph a few months after treatment (Fig. 4). One simple observation by a resident led to the correct path of management.

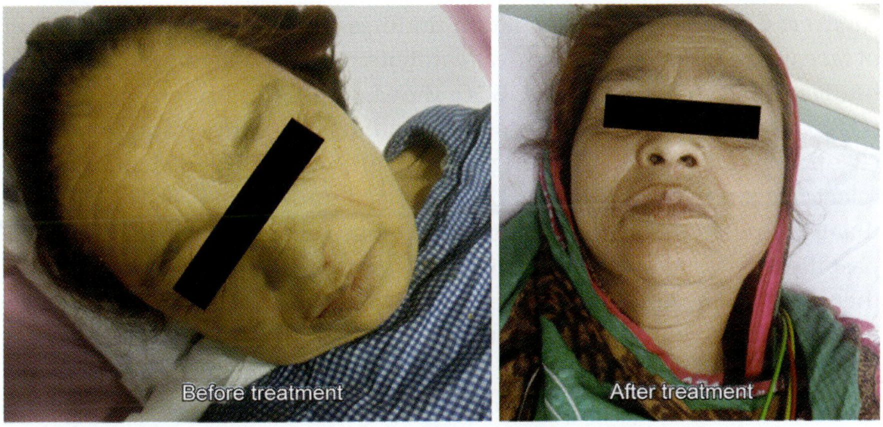

Fig. 4: The patient at presentation, and after a few months.

What is possibly is the observation and the diagnosis?

Pause and think before you click the answer:

Answer: Characteristic examination findings were yellowish discoloration of face with sparing of conjunctiva (carotenemia), myxedema, hypothermia, bradycardia, and drowsiness. ECG showed sinus bradycardia, long QT (QTc of 580 ms) and malignant ventricular premature complex (VPC) (R on T phenomenon) leading to multiple runs of ventricular flutter (electrical storm). Laboratory reports showed undetectable TSH (0.001 IU) that triggered investigations for central hypothyroidism. On further probing, past history revealed lactation failure 30 years back and amenorrhea since then. MRI brain showed empty sella as in **Case 2**. She was treated with high dose levothyroxine and corticosteroids. Patient showed dramatic clinical improvement with normalization of QTc interval and no further episodes of VT on follow-up. Sheehan syndrome led to electrical storm in this patient. Without identifying the underlying Sheehan syndrome, this patient could not have recovered.

Her ECG on follow-up is shown in **Figure 5**.

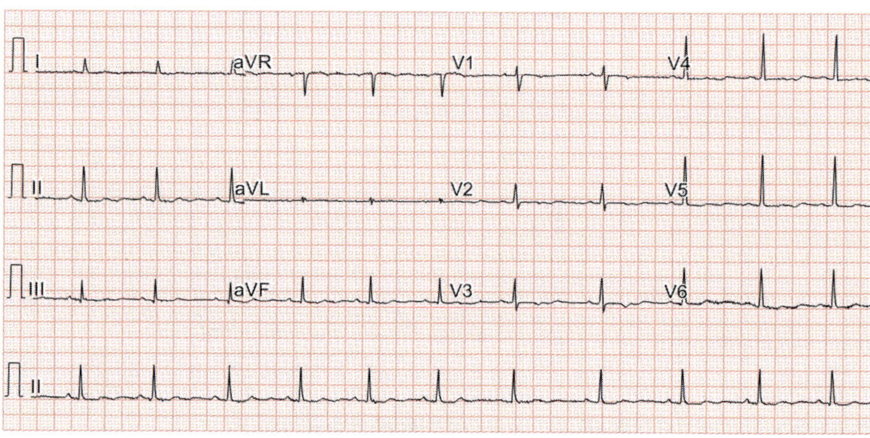

Fig. 5: ECG at follow-up.

Her hormone profile and MRI picture are shown below **(Table 1 and Figs. 6A to C)**.

TABLE 1: Hormone profile of the patient.

Hormone, unit	*Patient's value*	*Normal range*
Tri-iodothyronine (T3), ng/mL	0.23	0.58–1.59
Thyroxine (T4), µg/dL	1.27	4.86–11.72
Thyroid stimulating hormone, mIU/mL	00	0.35–4.94
Prolactin, ng/mL	3.3	5.18–26.53
Follicle stimulating hormone, mIU/mL	2.43	26.7–133.41
Luteinizing hormone, IU/mL	1.5	10.39–64.75
IGF-1, ng/mL	7.49	44–240
Fasting cortisol, µg/dL	4.0	5–25
ACTH, pg/mL	<1.0	6–76

(ACTH: adrenocorticotropic hormone; IGF-1: insulin-like growth factor 1)

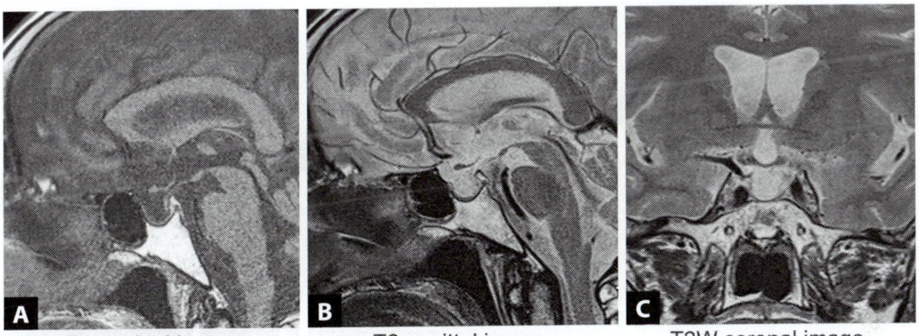

T1 sagittal image | T2 sagittal image | T2W coronal image

Figs. 6A to C: MRI showing atrophic anterior pituitary gland.

Learning points: These two rather exceptional cases **(Cases 2 and 3)** make an important point that reversible causes of cardiomyopathy must be sought before labeling any patient as dilated cardiomyopathy. Once a label is stuck, it is unlikely that on follow-up, the etiology will be discovered.

Furthermore, reversible causes of systolic muscle dysfunction should also be considered even in patients with "usual" dilated cardiomyopathy so that some clinical improvement might occur with the treatment of those factors even in patients of any type of dilated cardiomyopathy. This fact cannot be overemphasized.

(*Source:* Narang R, Reddy SS. Look says it all—Clinically recognizable electrical storm. Indian J Med Res. 2020;152(Suppl 1):S8-S9.)

Sidelights:

1. **What are the causes of polymorphic VT?**
2. **For the same degree of QT prolongation, Torsades de pointes is rarer with which causes of prolonged QT?**
3. **How to manage a patient found to have empty sella on a MRI done for doubtful syncope?**

(*Sidelights are food for thought—provided to increase your curiosity:* So as a rule, do not read these answers before you try to answer them yourself. The answers provided here are not intended to be exhaustive.)

Answer: Polymorphic VT may occur with prolong QT (typical Torsades de pointes tachycardia) or may occur with normal QT interval as in acute ischemic phase of myocardial infarction (MI) with ST segment elevations. In chronic coronary artery disease (CAD), polymorphic VT with normal QT interval may occur sometimes from Purkinje fibers and that VT has a short coupling interval. Such polymorphic VTs are also seen in Brugada syndrome, idiopathic VF, or with short QT syndrome. The coupling interval initiating the VT is longer in Torsades and it is shorter in the other varieties described. Many of the polymorphic VTs with short coupling interval (<400 ms) respond to quinidine that is contraindicated in typical Torsades de pointes tachycardia.

- The QT prolongation with hypocalcemia, very rarely causes Torsades and Torsades is relatively less common with amiodarone also, as both of these lead to homogenous QT prolongation throughout the myocardium. Thus, with less heterogeneity of repolarization, ventricular arrhythmias are relatively rare.
- Empty sella is frequently found on MRI and in the absence of any symptoms it may be a benign finding. It is reported in 8–35% of neuroimaging studies. It might indicate a significant pituitary problem, or intracranial hypertension, but might be a benign finding without clinical implications. So, as always, clinical context is required for the interpretation of any of the tests.

CASE

4

Dilated Cardiomyopathy

"The pursuit of truth and beauty is a sphere of activity in which we are permitted to remain children all our lives."

—Albert Einstein

A 32-year-old man presented with progressively worsening exertional breathlessness of 3 months duration. On examination, there was tachycardia, tachypnea, tender hepatomegaly, pedal edema, and elevated jugular venous pressure. Auscultation revealed bilateral basal crepitations, left ventricular (LV) third heart sound, and a pan-systolic murmur at the apex suggestive of mitral regurgitation (MR). His X-ray, ECG, and echo are shown in **Figures 1 to 3**. The echo showed severe LV dysfunction with ejection fraction (EF) 20% and an apical thrombus **(Videos 1 and 2)**.

Video 1 Video 2

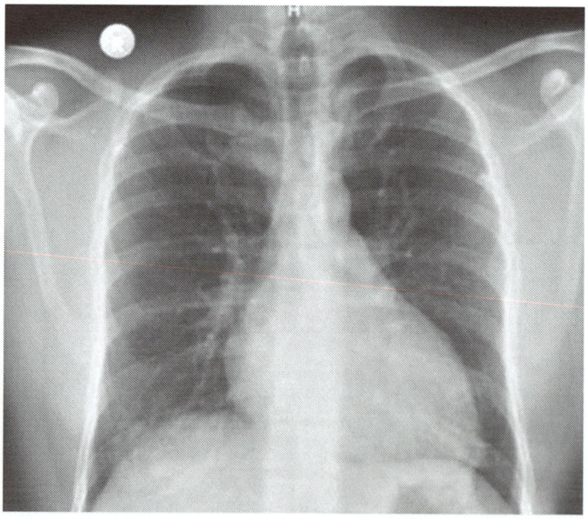

Fig. 1: Chest X-ray at presentation.

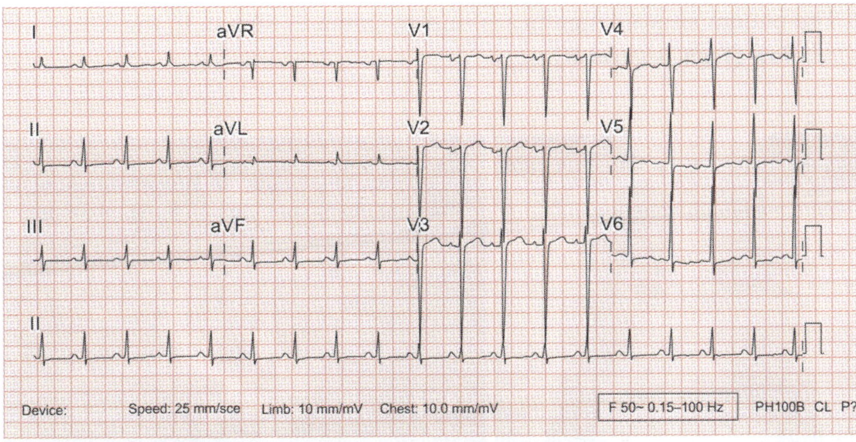

Fig. 2: ECG at presentation.

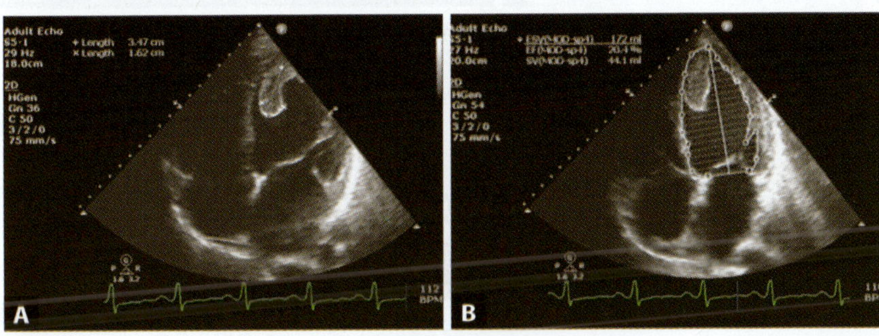

Figs. 3A and B: Two-dimensional echocardiography image in apical four-chamber view. (A) Biventricular dilation with a large apical left ventricular thrombus; (B) Severe left ventricular dysfunction with an ejection fraction of 20.4% (by Simpsons' method).

The patients photograph is shown in **Figure 4**.

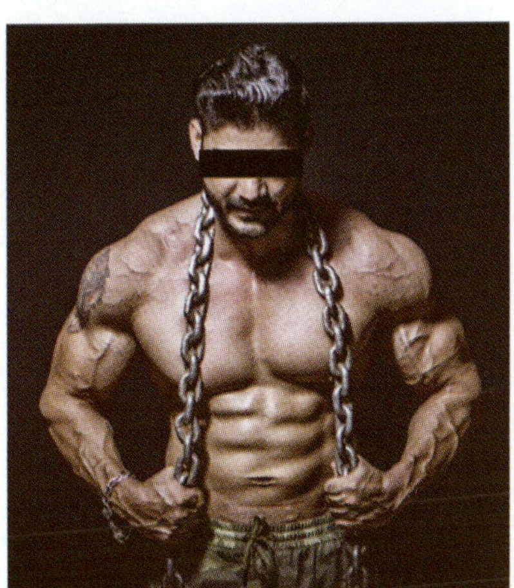

Fig. 4: Patient's photograph 3 months prior.

The patient showed significant improvement as shown in the X-ray and echo below **(Figs. 5A and B)**.

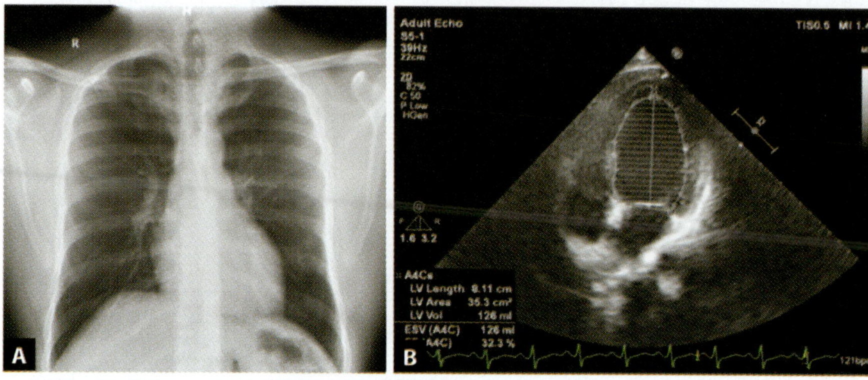

Figs. 5 and B: (A) X-ray after treatment; (B) Echo after treatment.

The LVEF on echo had improved to 32% (by Simpsons' method) **(Video 3)**.

Video 3

The improvement was possible due to a piece of information in history. In the context, what could be that history?

Pause and think before you click the answer:

Answer: The patient had acute onset heart failure after starting intravenous mephentermine as a physical performance enhancing substance. Mephentermine is structurally similar to methamphetamine and was used as a stimulant before work out. He initially did not disclose this history, but a friendly persistent questioning revealed that patients has used testosterone esters, drostanolone, and nandrolone (300 mg, 200 mg, and 150 mg intramuscularly daily, respectively) for last 2 years. These drugs were taken in cycles of 45 days followed by a drug-free period of 6 months before the next cycle. He started using 30 mg mephentermine intravenously daily for last 3 months that coincided with the symptoms. Though he has taken anabolic steroids for quite sometime, the symptoms coincided with the use of mephentermine. Stopping mephentermine resulted in marked resolution of cardiac function. Anabolic steroid-induced ventricular dysfunction is known, but mephentermine-induced cardiomyopathy was reported for the first time. This also reminds us of catecholamine induced cardiac systolic dysfunction that occurs in patients with Takotsubo cardiomyopathy, pheochromocytoma, and other situations with high sympathetic drive.

(*Source:* Singal AK, Deepti S, Sharma G, Kothari SS. Herculean mistake: mephentermine associated cardiomyopathy. Phys Sports med. 2021; 49(1):116-22.)

Learning points: Catecholamine-induced cardiac systolic dysfunction is seen in takotsubo cardiomyopathy, pheochromocytoma, and is an experimental model to induce cardiomyopathy in animals.

Catecholamine-induced cardiomyopathy, might have QT prolonged on ECG (though isoprenaline is used to treat prolong QT). This patient's ECG (Fig. 1) also showed mildly prolonged QT that was not realized at admission.

(Anabolic steroid-induced myocardial dysfunction was suspected from the patients profile, but it was not immediately apparent as the patient denied the use of performance enhancing drugs highlighting the importance of art of history taking that is not same as digitized information gathering.)

If you found the above case too easy; try this one.

Case 4A: Bonus Case

In searching for a treatable cause of ventricular systolic dysfunction, we have to be sensitive to any possible cue. The ECG below **(Figs. 6A and B)** is from a child with severe ventricular dysfunction that resolved with some treatment. Does it provide any clue?

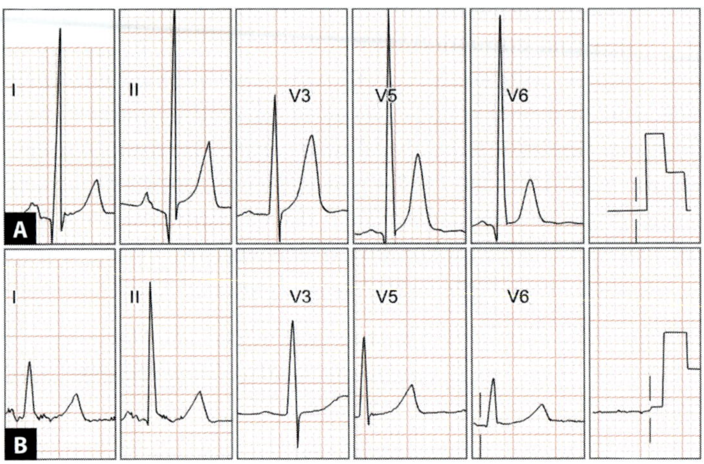

Figs. 6A and B: The ECG of the patient before and after (lower panel) treatment. (*Source:* Fu L, Huang M, Chen S. Korean Circ J. 2013;43(12):785-92.)

And another similar patient ***(Fig. 7)****:*

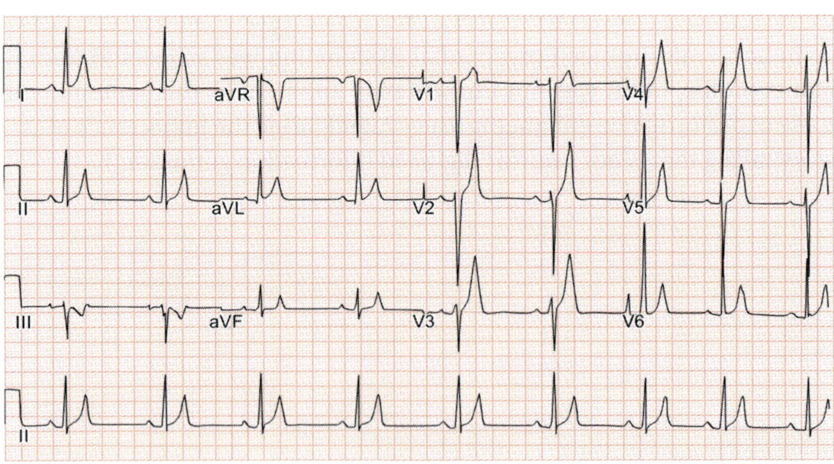

Fig. 7: ECG.
(*Source:* Tomlinson S, Atherton J, Prasad S. Case Rep Cardiol. 2018;2018:3232105.)

Do these ECGs suggest a diagnosis in which case the ventricular function might improve with supplementation?

Pause and think before you click the answer:

Answer: Primary carnitine deficiency is a treatable cause of LV dysfunction. The ECG show LV hypertrophy (LVH), tall-peaked T waves and short QT interval. Many such cases have been published. There is some evidence to suggest that cardiolipotoxicity of accumulated lipids cause abnormality in potassium channels that accounts for short QT interval and arrythmia (even acquired carnitine deficiency might show similar ECG changes). The sensitivity, and specificity of this ECG findings for the diagnosis of carnitine deficiency, however, remains unclear. Resolution of ventricular dysfunction has been described with carnitine supplementation in such cases.

Sidelights:

1. **What is cobalt cardiomyopathy?**
2. **ECGs of patients with prolong QT and ventricular dysfunction are shown in Figures 8 and 9. But it is not due to catecholamines. What could this be? Does the shape of QT prolongation provide any clue?**

(*Sidelights are food for thought—provided to increase your curiosity:* So as a rule, do not read these answers before you try to answer them yourself. The answers provided here are not intended to be exhaustive.)

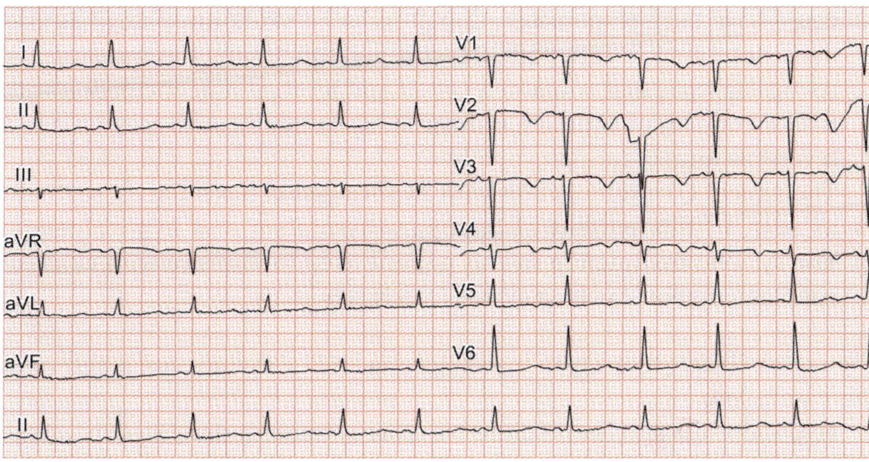

Fig. 8: ECG showing prolong QT interval in a patient with ventricular dysfunction. (*Source:* Baqi DH, Ahmed SF, Baba HO, Fattah FH, Salih AM, Ali RM, et al. Ann Med Surg (Lond). 2022;77:103572.)

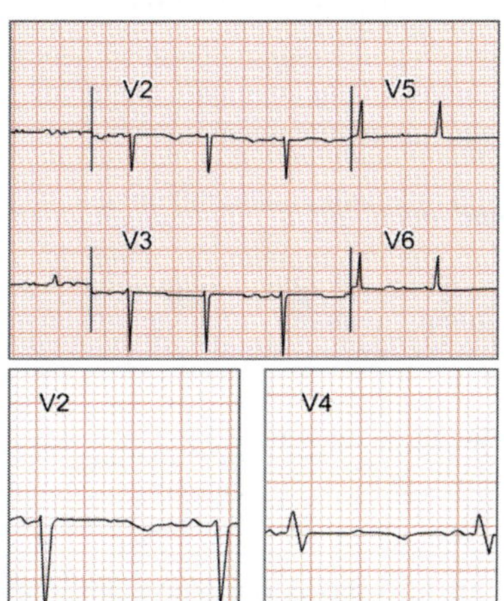

Fig. 9: ECG showing prolong QT interval in a patient with ventricular dysfunction. (*Source:* Lam J, Maragaño P, Lépez B, Vásquez L. Rev Med Chil. 2007;135(3):359-64.)

Answer: Cobalt-induced ventricular dysfunction was seen in beer drinkers cardiomyopathy in Canada at a time when cobalt was added in the beer. The cardiomyopathy was characterized by rapid onset of heart failure, pericardial effusion, lack of arrythmias, polycythemia, and goiter. Most of these patients were nutritionally deficient and multiple causes could have been responsible. Cobalt-induced cardiomyopathy has also been described in rare patients with malfunctioning hip implants (of particular types that contained cobalt and leeched it in circulation with malfunctioning prosthesis). Industrial exposure to cobalt may lead to a reversible form of cardiomyopathy.

- The typical QT prolongation with hypocalcemia has a flat ST segment as seen in this patient of hypoparathyroidism and hypocalcemia. The systolic dysfunction in this patient used to improve with calcium supplementation. Such an event is rarely reported.

Even more clearer shape with hypocalcemia and LV dysfunction is shown in this case below.

Hypocalcemia and heart failure are more commonly described in infants and children. Neonates in particular are more dependent on calcium for myocardial contraction and several cases of hypocalcemic heart failure have been described in them. Below is an example. In neonates, the QoT interval, i.e., interval from Q waves to onset of T wave is prolonged with hypocalcemia **(Fig. 10)**. Shown below an old record of an infant who improved markedly with calcium within 10 days **(Figs. 11A and B)**.

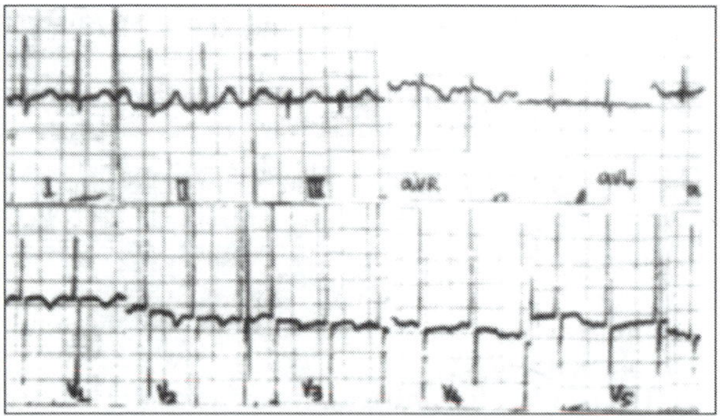

Fig. 10: ECG showing prolong QoT interval.

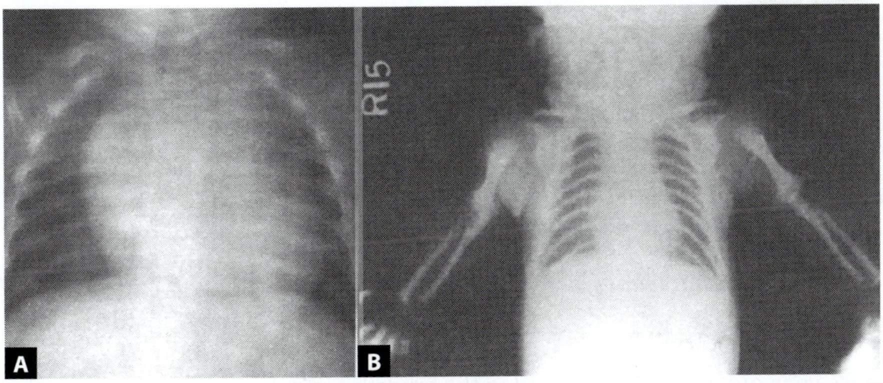

Figs. 11A and B: Chest X-ray before (A) and (B) after calcium replacement.
(Source: Gulati S, Bajpai A, Juneja R, Kabra M, Bagga A, Kalra V. Hypocalcemic heart failure masquerading as dilated cardiomyopathy. Indian J Pediatr. 2001;68(3):287-90.)

The ECG in infants must be viewed carefully to pick up a prolonged corrected QoT interval (Fig. 10), because it could be missed due to tachycardia.

CASE

5

Complete Heart Block

"It's not what you look at that matters, it's what you see."

—Henry David Thoreau

A 65-year-old woman presented to the emergency room with syncope earlier in the day. She had recurrent episodes of giddiness, lethargy, generalized weakness, and anorexia for the past 6 months. She also complained of severe constipation for the past 1 year with a reduction in stool frequency to once to twice per week. She had mild systemic hypertension for which she took medications irregularly.

On presentation in the emergency room, she was fully conscious, with a pulse rate of 30 beats/min and a blood pressure of 150/80 mm Hg. She had an otherwise unremarkable cardiovascular examination. Fecoliths were palpable on abdominal examination. ECG revealed complete heart block with a narrow QRS escape at a rate of 33 beats/min with a QT and QTc intervals of 520 ms and 426 ms, respectively **(Fig. 1)**. The trop I was negative and echo showed concentric left ventricular hypertrophy (LVH) and normal ventricular systolic function. The serum sodium and potassium levels were normal.

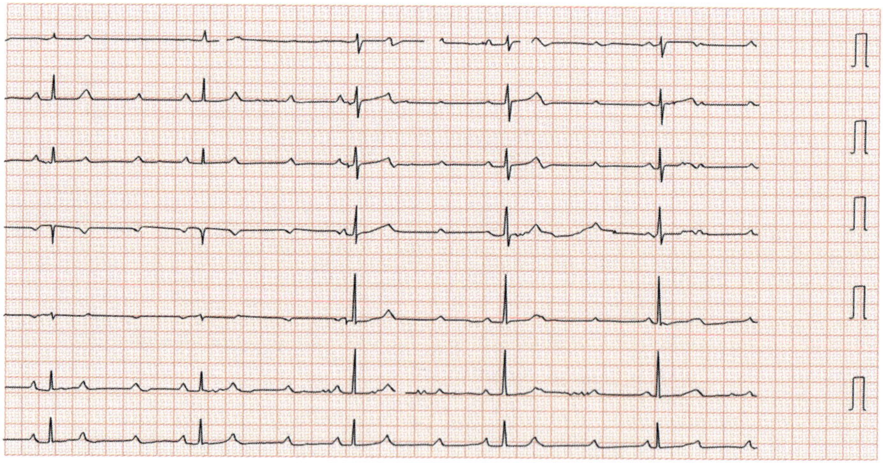

Fig. 1: ECG showing complete heart block.

She had a temporary pacemaker placed. After some treatment, the repeat ECG is shown in Figure 2. She did not require a pacemaker on follow-up. Can you reflect on the given story and guess the possible causes of reversible complete heart block in this patient? How would you investigate this patient?

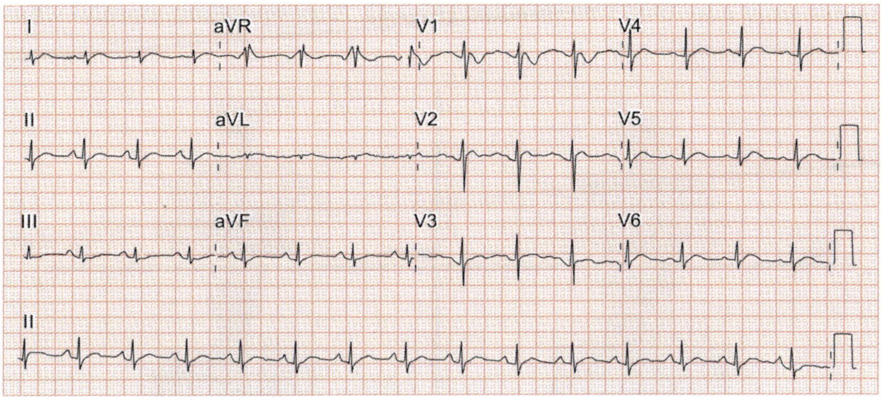

Fig. 2: ECG after treatment.

Pause and think before you click the answer:

Answer: The presence of narrow QRS complex was unusual for the typical sclerodegenerative complete heart block that we commonly encounter at this age. The serum calcium was 17 mg% and further evaluation confirmed the diagnosis of a parathyroid adenoma on sestamibi scan **(Fig. 3)**. The heart block disappeared as the serum calcium was lowered with fluid and intravenous furosemide and reappeared as the calcium levels increase. The parathyroid adenoma was resected **(Fig. 4)**. After operation, normal sinus rhythm was established.

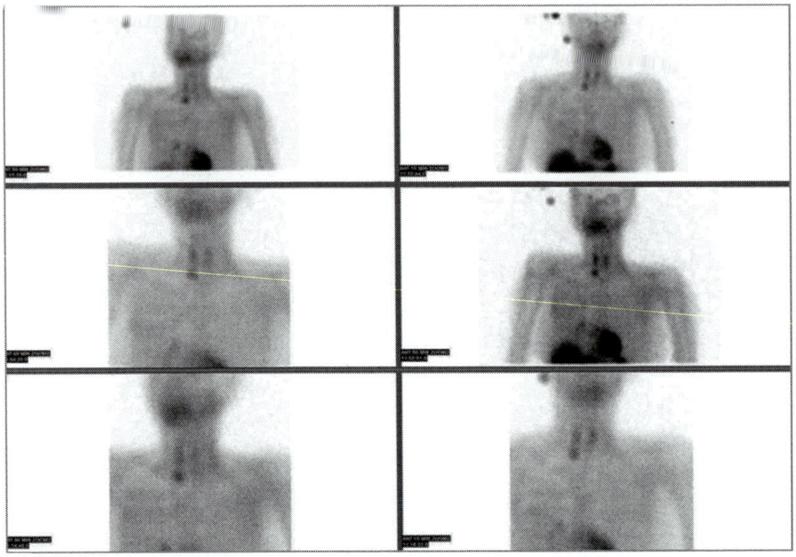

Fig. 3: Sestamibi scan showed right inferior parathyroid nodule.

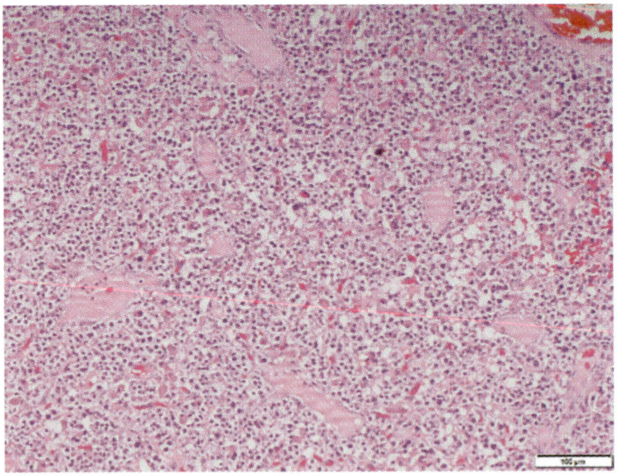

Fig. 4: Parathyroid adenoma.
(*Source:* Ramakumar V, Kothari SS, Seth S, Kumar S. Reversible complete heart block due to hypercalcaemia. BMJ Case Rep. 2021;14(1):e238537.)

Learning points: Hypercalcemia might cause reversible complete heart block. As seen in this case, heart block might occur even in the absence of typical ECG signs of hypercalcemia such as QT shortening or epsilon waves. Similar cases have also been reported in the literature.

Sidelights:

1. **Narrate other causes of reversible complete heart block.**
2. **What is the difference between J wave and Epsilon wave?**
3. **What are the causes of Epsilon wave?**
4. **How do we treat hypermagnesemia?**

(*Sidelights are food for thought—provided to increase your curiosity:* So as a rule, do not read these answers before you try to answer them yourself. The answers provided here are not intended to be exhaustive.)

Answer: Reversible complete heart block frequently occurs with inferior myocardial infarction (MI) and in prinzmetal angina. It may be seen due to drugs like B blockers, calcium blockers, antiarrhythmics, tricyclic antidepressant, digoxin, herbal medications, electrolyte disturbances like hyperkalemia, hypercalcemia; hypo- and hyperthyroidism, infectious myocarditis like Lymes disease, viral myocarditis, and diphtheria. A less well recognized cause is from vagotonia (vagotonia might give rise to mobitz type 3 block as well and a long pause. Associated sinus bradycardia may be a clue). Rheumatic fever does not cause complete heart block (only very rare case reports described). Some of the drug-induced heart block might require permanent pacing even, as there may be significant conduction disturbance unmasked by the drug.

- J wave and epsilon wave both represent the phenomenon occurring at or near the end of QRS. These waves may result either from a prolongation of depolarization in some areas, or a gradient in the epicardium to endocardium during repolarization in some areas. Epsilon waves are sharper, smaller, and higher frequency signals seen mostly in the right-sided leads whereas J waves are rounded, lower frequency slightly larger, and seen in lateral and inferior leads. J waves are seen with hypothermia, hypercalcemia, early repolarization syndrome, normal variant, LVH, subarachnoid hemorrhage, idiopathic ventricular fibrillation (VF), and Brugada syndrome. Case reports of J waves in MI and Takotsubo cardiomyopathy have been described. Epsilon waves are typically seen in arrhythmogenic right ventricular cardiomyopathy (ARVC), Brugada syndrome, right ventricular infarction, posterior infarction, sarcoidosis, or other infiltration on the epicardium.
- The question is asked only to remind that calcium and magnesium may be considered as physiological antagonist and hypermagnesemia is treated with IV calcium if required. Conversely, hypokalemia and hypocalcemia are not effectively corrected until serum magnesium is replenished to normal levels. Thus ECG of hypomagnesemia may present as ECG of hyperkalemia as potassium cannot get into the cell and high extra- versus intracellular gradient may simulate an ECG of hyperkalemia. Such clinical examples are rarely recorded.

If you already knew all that then see an example of functional atrioventricular (AV) block ECG below (Figs. 5 to 7).

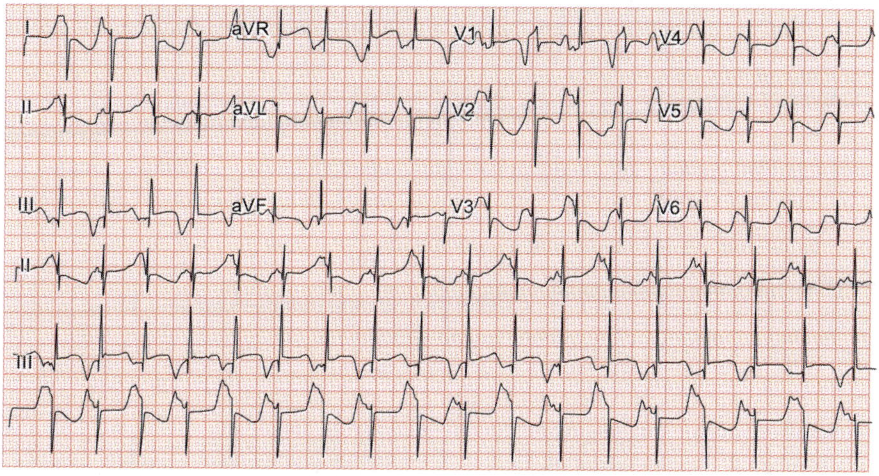

Fig. 5: ECG sinus rhythm 1:1 conduction.

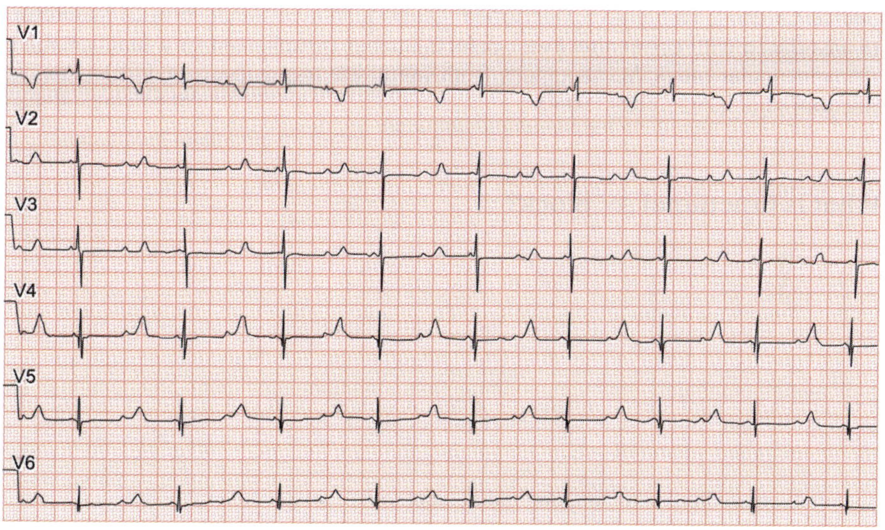

Fig. 6: ECG with 2:1 AV block with decrease in sinus rate.

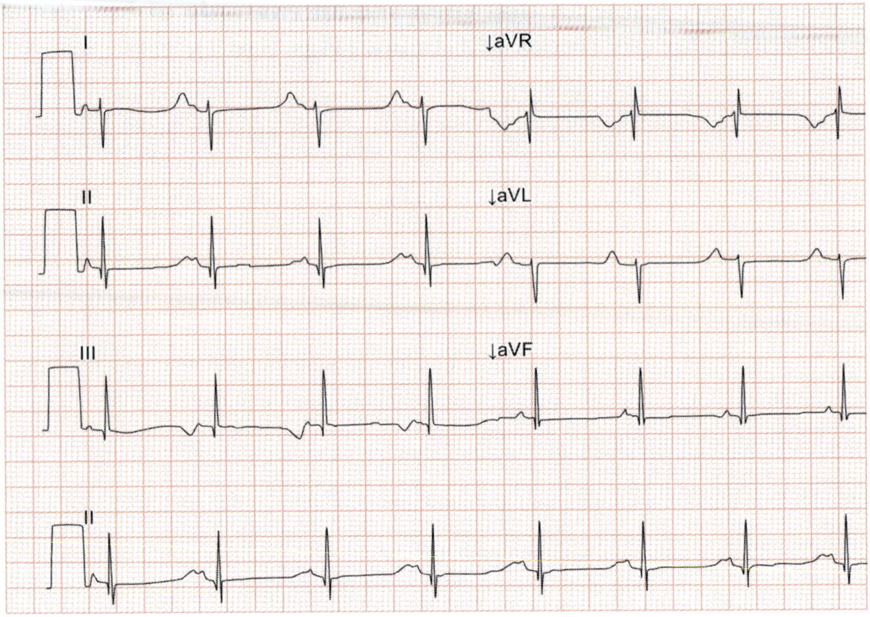

Fig. 7: ECG with 1:1 conduction.
(*Source:* Caruso E, Farruggio S, Guccione P. Calmodulin mutation in long QT syndrome 15 associated with congenital heart defects further complicated by a functional 2:1 atrioventricular block: Management from foetal life to postpartum. Indian Pacing Electrophysiol J. 2024;24(3):150-4.)

What is functional AV block?

Answer: ECG of a newborn shows prolonged QT interval and heart rate of 100 in the top panel, (QTC 640 ms). As the sinus rate decreases and the QT interval further prolonged (QTc 800 ms), there is a functional 2:1 AV block since the P wave reaches the ventricle that has not yet recovered due to long refractoriness (prolonged QT interval). With esmolol, the QT interval shortens somewhat and there is sinus rhythm again (Fig. 7). Hence, one can see that the block is due to prolonged refractoriness and not structural in this instance. Note the P wave engulfed by the T in case of 2:1 block. The block is not in the node, but somewhere in the Purkinje system or the myocardium.

They might have true AV block from the disease in the conduction system as well, when the P would not be conducted despite being beyond the T waves.

Patients with congenital long QT syndrome with conduction heart block (CHB) generally have more Torsades and poorer prognosis. They should be paced and should receive beta-blockers. The QT interval shortens with pacing.

And after functional, and metabolic cause of AV block, look at an organic cause of conduction system disease. The ECG shown below (Fig. 8) is from a 17-year-old girl with recent history of giddiness and atypical chest pain.

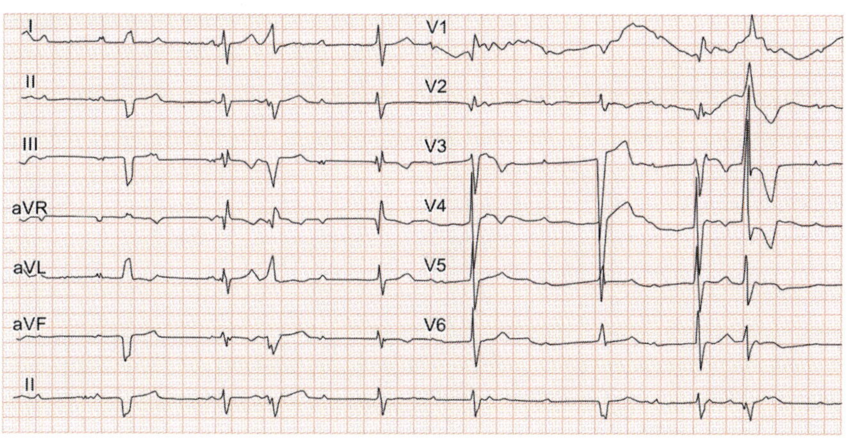

Fig. 8: ECG.

Her Echo are shown in **Videos 1 and 2**.

Video 1 **Video 2**

What is the cause of the conduction system disease?

Pause and think before you click the answer:

Answer: The interesting echo videos show a mass in the interventricular septum that is expansile and also contains cavity and thrombus. It is a sinus of Valsalva aneurysm burrowing into the interventricular septum. The 3D volume rendered CT shows the aneurysm very well **(Fig. 9)**.

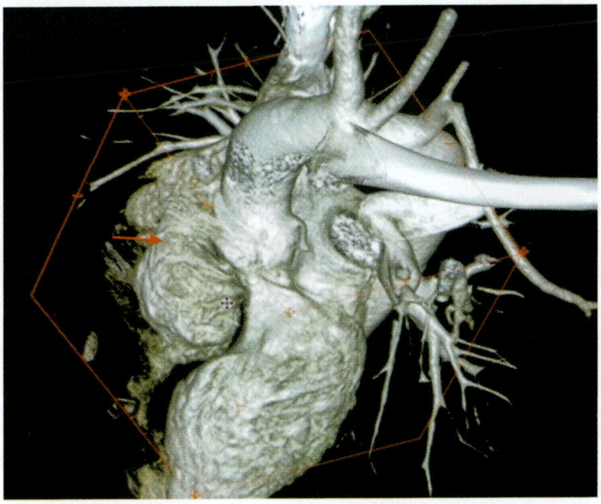

Fig. 9: The 3D volume rendered CT shows the right sinus of Valsalva aneurysm into the ventricular septum (red arrow).

CASE

6

Stroke in the Young

"The eyes do not see what the mind does not know."

—Anonymous

A 35-year-old man had acute onset weakness in right side of the body and aphasia. The patient was asymptomatic prior to this episode. A MRI showed acute middle cerebral artery infarct. There were no previous episodes of arterial or venous thrombosis, or a family history of similar disorders. The patient enjoyed good health and had no medical illness except an atrial septal defect (ASD) operated at 4 years of age. The ECG and chest X-ray were normal. His hemoglobin was 17 g with normal total and differential counts, and normal platelets. No definite abnormality was found by the hematologists who did not register that the oximetric saturation was 88%. Thus the polycythemia was secondary to arterial desaturation and did not need hematologic investigations actually. Clinical examination showed clubbing, and normal cardiac examination. One of his investigation is shown in the **Video 1**. The image of the same is also shown in **Figure 1**.

Video 1

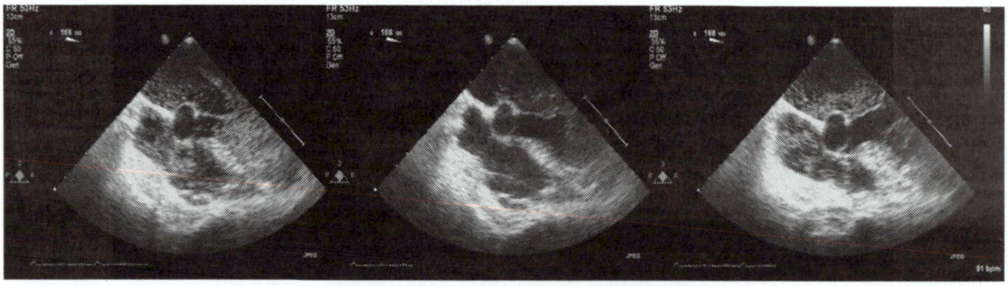

Fig. 1: Contrast echo images.

What is the diagnosis?

Pause and think before you click the answer:

Answer: The patient had an ASD operated at the age of 4 years. Though the details were not available, this history coupled with the hypoxia on oximeter was highly suspicious of the fact that the polycythemia could be related to ASD closure. In the echo room a contrast from the upper limb was normal, but the contrast injection from the lower limb streamed into left atrium (LA) diagnosing a known complication of ASD surgery of inadvertently directing the inferior vena cava (IVC) flow into the LA. This rare complication occurs when sutures mistakenly direct IVC flow to LA. It is usually seen when the eustachian valve is included in the repair, or when a low lying ASD's inferior edge is missed and IVC overrides the residual defect.

In this patient, subsequently a cardiac catheterization from lower limb also showed IVC blood streaming into the LA (**Video 2**). The patient was reoperated successfully.

Video 2

(*Source:* Desai M, Talwar S, Kothari SS, Jagia P, Airan B. Inferior vena cava to left atrium shunt presenting with polycythemia and stroke three decades following closure of atrial septal defect. Congenit Heart Dis. 2013;8(4):E102-5.)

Learning points: Polycythemia with hypoxemia does not require hematological investigations. Surgical closure of ASD might direct IVC to LA, even though it sounds unconvincing. Apart from this rare but known complication of ASD surgical closure, a prominent eustachian valve in patients with an ASD/patent foramen ovale (PFO) might direct the IVC blood to LA and this right-to-left shunt might be dependent on posture causing platypnea-orthodeoxia (patient has desaturation and discomfort on sitting up and feels better on lying down, sometimes diagnosed as functional or psychogenic. >5% change in the saturation with posture is generally accepted as suggestive of the syndrome).

Sidelights:

1. **What are the other causes of platypnea-orthodeoxia?**
2. **What are the causes of cyanosis and structurally normal heart?**

(*Sidelights are food for thought—provided to increase your curiosity:* So as a rule, do not read these answers before you try to answer them yourself. The answers provided here are not intended to be exhaustive.)

Answer: Platypnea-orthodeoxia occurs with right-to-left shunting through an ASD/PFO that is enhanced due to anatomic factors such as a large eustachian valve, dilated aorta, aortic aneurysms compressing and altering the position of PFO/ASD, kyphoscoliosis, and after pneumonectomy. The saturation might drop <90% on standing and improves with lying down. It might also occur without an ASD in patients with pulmonary AV fistula in the basal region, or in hepatopulmonary syndrome with microscopic AV fistulae that are more in the basal region. Severe ventilation-perfusion mismatch in interstitial lung disease, chronic obstructive airway disease, or even in a pneumonia that is affected due to position might also cause platypnea-orthodeoxia without an intracardiac shunting.

- Cyanosis with structurally normal heart occurs in pulmonary AV fistula, methemoglobinemia and few other conditions that you know! (Read later).

Bonus echo:

The **Video 3** shows contrast echo again.
Where is the injection given? What does it show?

Video 3

Answer: The saline bubble contrast from the left arm fills the coronary sinus first that drains mainly to right atrium. However, partial unroofing in coronary sinus leads to contrast bubbles seen in LA and going to LV.

(*Source:* Gupta SK, Shetkar SS, Ramakrishnan S, Kothari SS. Saline Contrast Echocardiography in the Era of Multimodality Imaging—Importance of "Bubbling It Right". Echocardiography. 2015;32(11):1707-19.)

CASE

7

Atrial Septal Defect with Cyanosis

"Everything should be made as simple as possible, but not simpler."
—Albert Einstein

A 16-year-old boy presented with exertional fatigue for last 1 year. He was noticed to have mild clubbing and oximeter showed a saturation of 88%. The chest X-ray and ECG were normal. There was an atrial septal defect (ASD) on echo shunting right-to-left, but no cause for the right-to-left shunting was identified. There was no evidence of pulmonary hypertension on examination or echocardiography. The echo are shown below **(Videos 1 to 3)**.

Video 1 Video 2 Video 3

What is the diagnosis and the management?

Pause and think before you click the answer:

Answer: In an ASD, normally the shunt is left-to-right as the left atrial pressures are higher than the right atrium, and the right ventricle is more compliant than the left ventricle. This patient has smaller right ventricle, no tricuspid valve stenosis, but contrast goes from right to the left atrium (Videos 1 and 2). On close scrutiny, a membrane in right atrium is identified (Video 3) that was responsible for a right ventricular hypoplasia and a right-to-left shunt (cor triatriatum dexter). Removal of the membrane and closure of ASD, [usually accompanied with a superior vena cava (SVC)—pulmonary artery connection to unload the right ventricle, i.e., one and a half ventricle repair] is the treatment.

Learning points: In a patient with ASD, the presence of cyanosis does not necessarily mean that the patient has Eisenmenger syndrome.

Sidelights: What are the prerequisites for one and a half ventricle repair?

(*Sidelights are food for thought—provided to increase your curiosity:* So as a rule, do not read these answers before you try to answer them yourself. The answers provided here are not intended to be exhaustive.)

Answer: In corrective cardiac surgery, if the right ventricle is smaller, the right ventricle preload is decreased by diverting the SVC directly to the pulmonary artery and leaving the right ventricle with only inferior vena cava (IVC) flow to be pumped to the lungs. Thus doing a Glenn operation in addition to whatever is the primary problem is called as a one and a half repair. For SVC flow to traverse the lungs without a pulsatile force, the pulmonary vascular resistance must be low, pulmonary artery size should be adequate, and left ventricular function should be normal. If the tricuspid z score (that correlates with RV size generally is >–2), the RV can accommodate the systemic blood flow (some people have even gone as far as –4 z also, and only an additional small ASD as a vent instead of one and a half ventricle repair might be done).

See another patient having ASD and cyanosis—

Case 7A: Atrial Septal Defect with Cyanosis

A 10-year-old girl was referred for cyanosis, breathlessness, and fatigue of 2 years duration. On examination, she had cardiomegaly and was in congestive heart failure. There were no murmurs. Her ECG and chest X-ray are shown in **Figures 1 and 2**. Other routine tests were normal except hemoglobin of 17 gm/dL. The echo is shown below **(Videos 4 and 5)**. The ASD was shunting right-to-left, but in contrast to the previous case there was no right ventricle hypoplasia. What is the diagnosis?

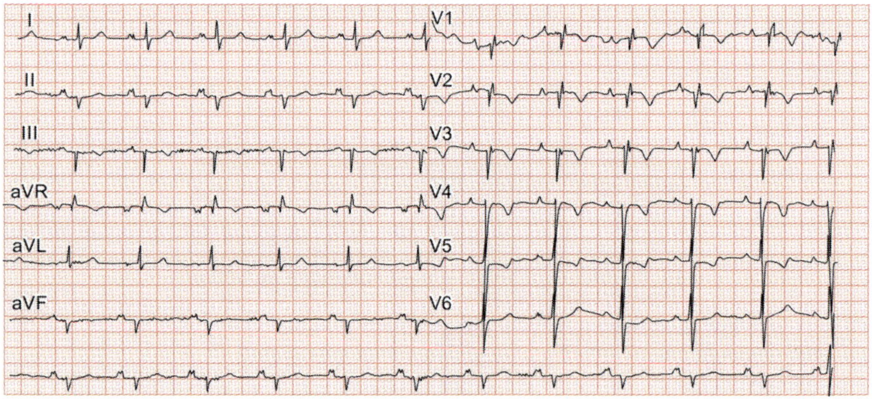

Fig. 1: ECG.

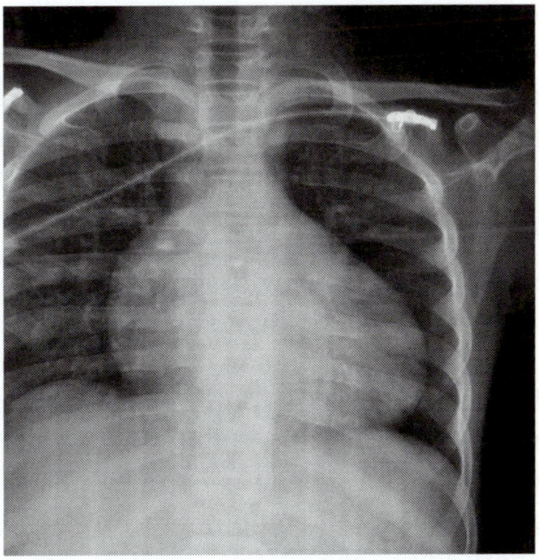

Fig. 2: Chest X-ray.

Video 4 **Video 5**

Pause and think before you click the answer:

Answer: The presence of heart failure should have alerted the clinicians that they are dealing with something sinister. Though there is no significant pulmonary arterial hypertension, the ECH showed severe right ventricular dysfunction. The patient had biventricular cardiomyopathy with more severe RV dysfunction than the left ventricular dysfunction, and therefore the ASD was shunting right-to-left. Did you notice the outpouching in the RV on echo?

Learning points: Thus when faced with a patient who has an ASD and is shunting right-to-left, several possibilities should be kept in mind.

- ASD with pulmonary hypertension and Eisenmenger syndrome is the obvious diagnosis. But if the pulmonary artery pressures are not significantly raised, then some other interesting possibilities are there.
- Total anomalous pulmonary venous connections may present in the adults and might have only mild pulmonary arterial hypertension (PAH).
- Unroofed coronary sinus (complete or partial) is easily diagnosed by a saline contrast echo from the left arm where contrast would first appear in the left atrium if the coronary sinus is unroofed.
- Streaming of SVC or IVC blood in sinus venosus ASD may cause some right-to-left shunt due to the override of SVC or IVC over the sinus venosus ASD.
- A large ASD like common atrium might have some desaturation due to common mixing.
- A large eustachian valve might cause streaming toward LA.
- Associated anomalies such as Ebstein anomaly or significant pulmonary stenosis may be responsible in some cases.
- Isolated RV hypoplasia is often missed as a cause of right-to-left shunting ASD with normal PA pressure. Cor triatriatum dexter may be responsible in causing lack of RV development but isolated RV hypoplasia might occur without cor triatriatum dexter also.
- RV cardiomyopathy may be missed unless carefully seen. The RV cardiomyopathy may be isolated RV cardiomyopathy, or a biventricular cardiomyopathy with more severe RV involvement that might cause the right-to-left shunt. For example, RV endomyocardial fibrosis is occasionally seen to cause cyanosis and heart failure.
- Atrial flutter in a patient with ASD can give cyanosis during the flutter.
- Rarely, a pulmonary arteriovenous fistula may coexist as a cause of cyanosis in a patient with ASD, but the shunting in ASD in those cases should not be right-to-left.

Sometimes, the Eustachian valve might direct the flow into LA only in upright position causing platypnea-orthodeoxia and such a thing may be acquired, for example after pneumonectomy, or with aortic dilatation and aging; thus confusing the clinical picture. These patients would complain of dyspnea on getting up and might often be misdiagnosed as "functional".

The saturation in supine and upright position might give a clue as discussed in **Case 6**.

Shown below is an uncommon cause of ASD with cyanosis even when the ASD shunt is left-to-right 1.5:1 or more (Videos 6 and 7). Can you identify the cause?

Video 6 Video 7

Answer: The patient had ASD with 2:1 shunt and mild systemic desaturation. The tricuspid regurgitation jet through ASD (see frame by frame in Video 6) was responsible for mild cyanosis despite a left-to-right ASD. The pulmonary veins were fully saturated ruling out a lung disease.

Sidelights: What has migraine to do with a patent foramen ovale (PFO)/ASD?

(*Sidelights are food for thought—provided to increase your curiosity:* So as a rule, do not read these answers before you try to answer them yourself. The answers provided here are not intended to be exhaustive.)

Answer: Several studies have reported an association of PFO, especially larger right-to-left shunts or atrial septal aneurysms, in patients of migraine, and more often in patients of migraine with an aura. Controlled trials have not shown a statistically significant difference in migraine with a device closure, even though remarkable results are seen in some patients. Antiplatelet therapy alone has also been effective in ameliorating symptoms in some patients suggesting the role of platelets microemboli in the genesis of migraine. Conversely, new-onset migraine headaches after ASD device closure have also been reported in 1–7% of patients, and probably also underline the importance of microemboli in the genesis of migraine.

CASE

8

Postoperative Ventricular Dysfunction

"You cannot step in the same river twice,
For the waters are forever flowing around...."

—Heraclitus

A 20-year-old-girl had exertional dyspnea for last 5 years. She had an ejection systolic murmur and a low pitch diastolic murmur on chest examination. Her oximetric saturation was 95%. The chest X-ray and ECG are shown in **Figures 1 and 2**.

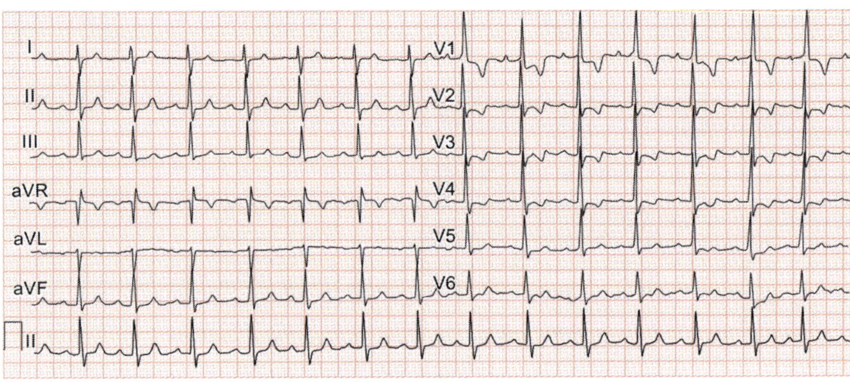

Fig. 1: ECG.

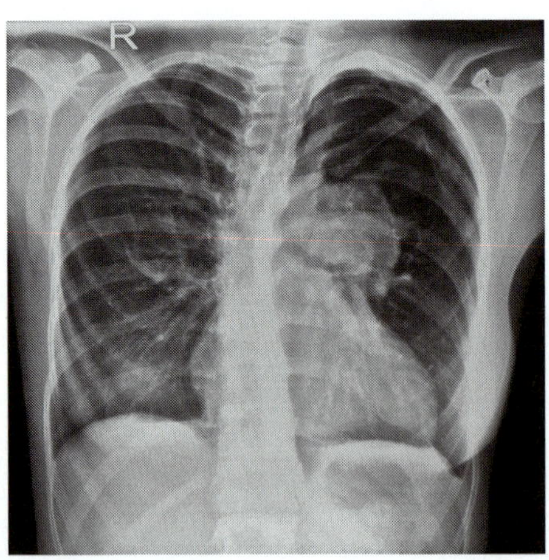

Fig. 2: Chest X-ray.

What is the diagnosis?

It is obvious that the patient has tetralogy of Fallot (TOF) with absent pulmonary valve as she had a pulmonary regurgitation murmur and right ventricular hypertrophy on ECG with markedly enlarged pulmonary arteries on chest X-ray. The echo showed a right ventricular outflow gradient of 70 mm Hg.

She underwent a corrective surgery with ventricular septal defect (VSD) closure and pulmonary valve replacement with a 25-mm bioprosthetic valve. Her postoperative course seemed alright. But on third day, she had hypotension and dyspnea and she had to be reintubated. The echo showed severe left ventricular (LV) dysfunction and an ejection fraction (EF) of 30%. The ECG immediately after operation **(Fig. 3)** and during the episode **(Fig. 4)** is shown below. The troponin levels were 3,590 ng/L. The ECG could be consistent with supraventricular tachycardia, but the patient did not improve even when the ECG showed sinus rhythm and was inotrope dependent.

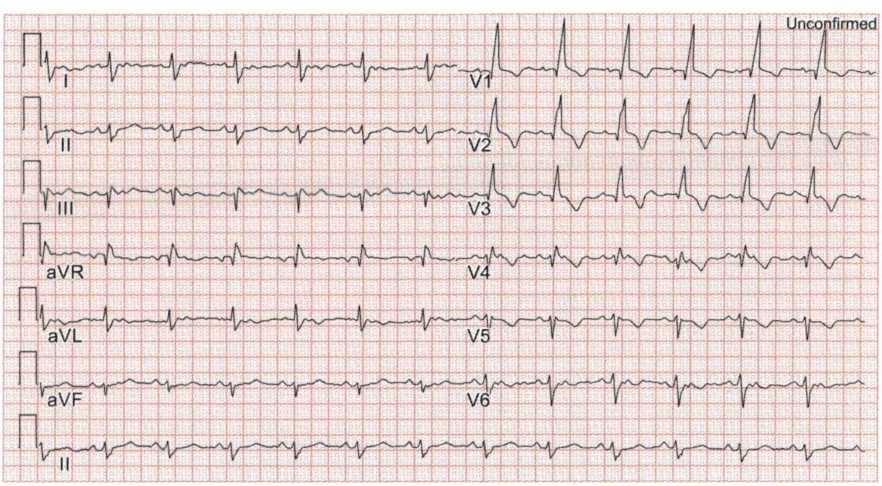

Fig. 3: Postoperative ECG.

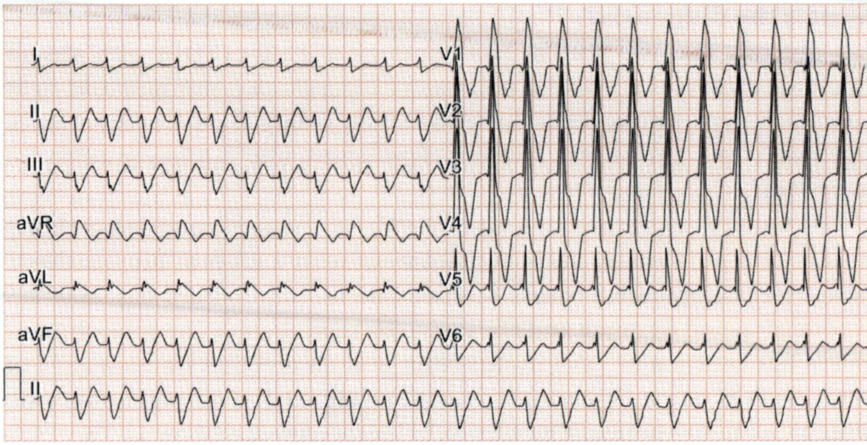

Fig. 4: ECG during the episode.

What possibilities should be considered?

Pause and think before you click the answer:

Answer: There could be several reasons for LV dysfunction in a postoperative patient. The patient had a smooth postoperative course and was extubated, thus cardiopulmonary bypass-related problems seem less likely. The context of the patient is important. The unusual course of the patient, the clinical diagnosis of absent pulmonary valve and the possibility of ischemia (due to raised troponins) made us wonder if the left main coronary artery (LMCA) might be compressed. Although the patient never had any symptoms previously, the preoperative CT did not show any bronchial or coronary compression, the patient was taken for a diagnostic coronary angiogram **(Video 1) (Fig. 5)**. The intravascular ultrasound (IVUS) also showed significant extrinsic compression of the LMCA **(Video 2)**.

A coronary angiogram done is shown below. And the IVUS withdrawal run from the LAD to LMCA is also shown.

Video 1 **Video 2**

A 4.5 × 18-mm drug-eluting stent was placed and postdilated with 5 × 18 noncompliant balloon with satisfactory result **(Fig. 6)**. She had quick improvement in that the ventricular premature complexes (VPCs) reduced and the blood pressures improved. She could be extubated after 6 hours. Her LV function recovered over a week and was completely normal on the follow-up after 1 month. Why did the LMCA compression manifested in the postoperative period is debatable. No pulmonary artery (PA) reduction was done as there were no signs of compression. According to some authors, PA reduction plasty should be done all cases where PA is larger than 4.5 mm (in any diagnosis) as, larger size PA can compress and change the takeoff angle of LMCA. Some alterations due to prosthetic pulmonary valve replacement (PVR) might account for the compression in postoperative setting, perhaps. In any case, it is important to correlate the findings and generate the right clinical context; and that has been the recurrent theme of clinical decision making.

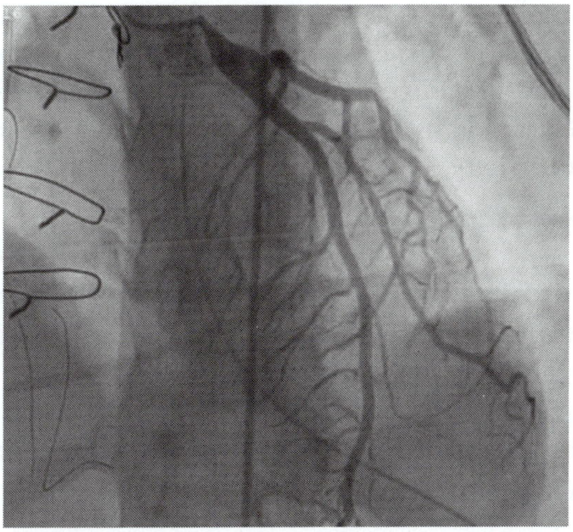

Fig. 5: Coronary angiography showing left main coronary artery (LMCA) compression.

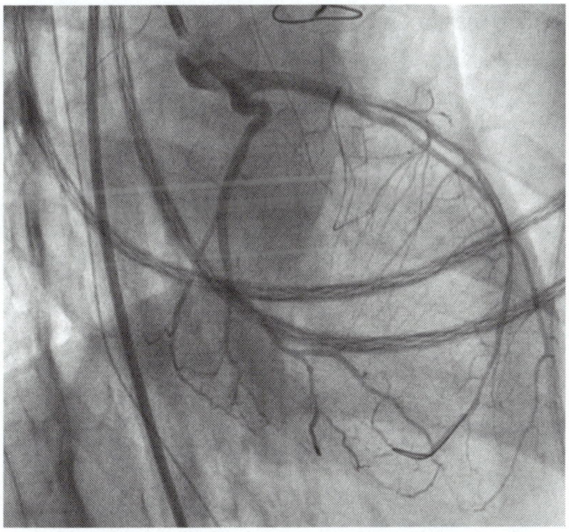

Fig. 6: Coronary angiography after left main coronary artery (LMCA) stenting.
(*Source:* Kothari SS, Sharma V, Patel K, Thakut G, Parikh R. Late post-operative cardiogenic shock from left main coronary compression in tetralogy of Fallot with absent pulmonary valve: a case report. Eur Heart J Case Rep. 2025 Apr 24;9(5):ytaf190. doi: 10.1093/ehjcr/ytaf190.)

Learning points: The LMCA compression is seen in patients with dilated pulmonary arteries (in about 6%) and may be missed unless a high index of suspicion is there. Such compression is more recognized in patients with primary pulmonary arterial hypertension, or Eisenmenger syndrome but may occur from PA dilatation due to any cause. PA size >40 mm possibly can alter the LMCA origin angle and may cause compression. A PA reduction plasty is recommended in TOF with absent pulmonary valve patients when PA size is >4.5 mm. The diagnosis in this patient is not completely secure, as the patient had LMCA compression discovered only after operation. Nevertheless, it is important to keep the right context in mind and hence the case is being shown here.

Sidelights: Coronary artery compression can occur from percutaneous pulmonary valve replacement and must be excluded by balloon interrogation before the valve is implanted.

When can the circumflex coronary artery compression occur during a cath lab procedure?

(*Sidelights are food for thought—provided to increase your curiosity:* So as a rule, do not read these answers before you try to answer them yourself. The answers provided here are not intended to be exhaustive.)

Answer: An anomalous circumflex from right ventricle coursing behind aorta might get compressed during an ASD device closure. This should be recognized during a preoperative echocardiography. Though not all patients with an anomalous circumflex coronary artery would have problem of compression with the device. So discretion is required, but it is important to be aware of this entity so that a sudden hypotension after ASD device closure is preempted.

CASE

9

Cardiogenic Shock in a Lady

"Medicine is a science of uncertainty and an art of probability."

—William Osler

A 48-year-old lady presented to emergency in cardiogenic shock. She had severe constricting chest pain while at work and had troponin markedly positive. She has no history of diabetes, hypertension, smoking, family history of premature coronary artery disease (CAD), or oral contraceptive use. Her ECG and echo are shown **Figure 1** and **videos 1 and 2**.

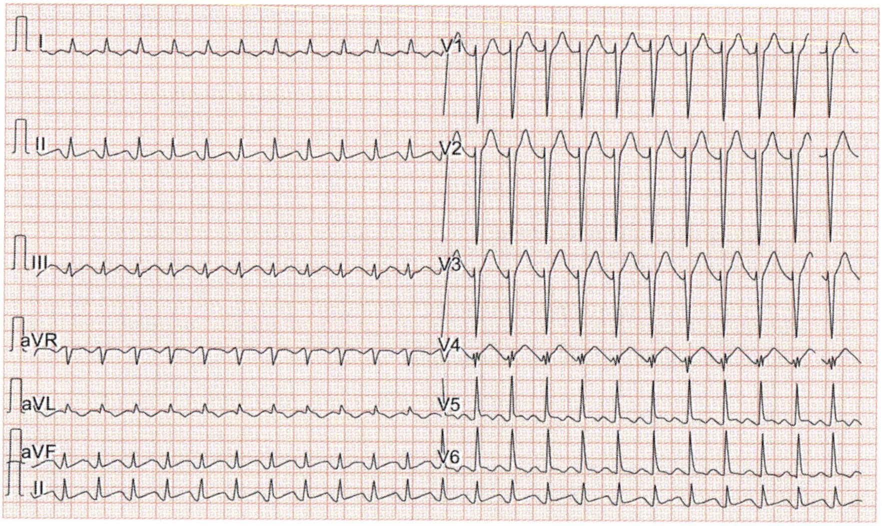

Fig. 1: ECG.

Video 1 **Video 2**

What would you like to consider?

Pause and think before you click the answer:

Answer: The lady had the symptoms after a physical fight with a male colleague at work! This history could offer a diagnosis of Takotsubo cardiomyopathy. Her coronary arteries were normal on angiography. She recovered well gradually. The repeat echo and ECG **(Fig. 2)** are shown below. The diffuse ST changes, prolongation of QT interval, and history supported the diagnosis. Of course, a coronary angiography would be needed even if you diagnosed Takotsubo cardiomyopathy.

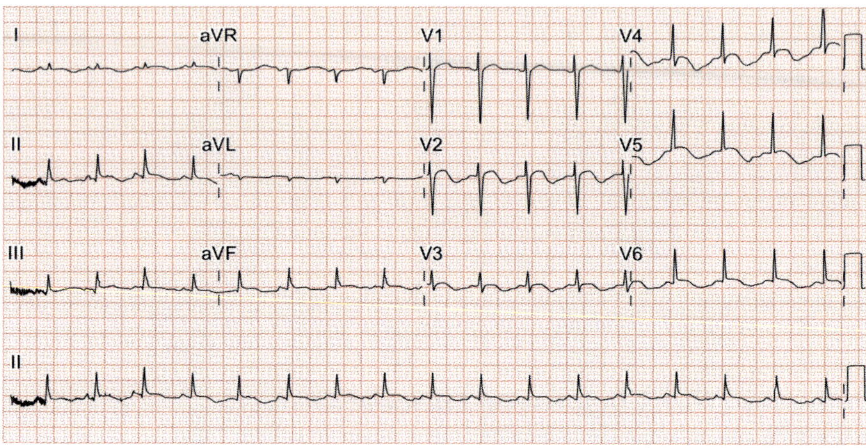

Fig. 2: The ECG at discharge.

Echo at discharge are shown in **Videos 3 and 4**.

Video 3 **Video 4**

Case 9A: A Bonus Reminder

A 27-year-old lady had episodic headaches and palpitation for last 3 years. She was discovered to have hypertension occasionally. Her father had a sudden death at the age of 34 years. On examination, she had blood pressure of 128/80 mm Hg. Her ECG and chest X-ray are shown below **(Figs. 3 and 4)**.

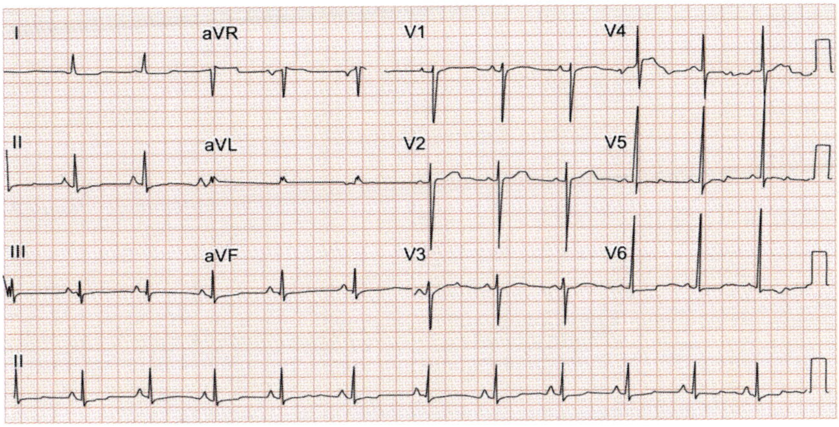

Fig. 3: ECG.

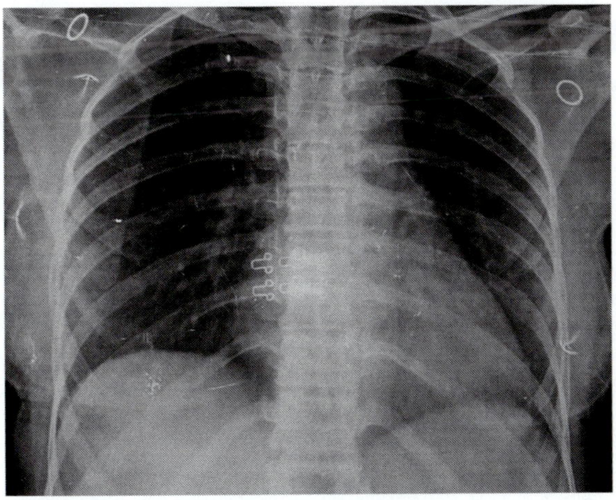

Fig. 4: Chest X-ray.

Routine investigations were normal.
Her echo is shown in **Videos 5 and 6**.

Video 5 **Video 6**

How would you like to investigate her?

Pause and think before you click the answer:

Answer: Though resting blood pressure was normal, the ECG and chest X-ray are suggestive of left ventricular (LV) hypertrophy. The echo shows mild LV dysfunction also. The family history of hypertension and early death is suspicious. She should be investigated for pheochromocytoma. The case is a reminder of that only; though patients with headache and hypertension rarely will have pheochromocytoma, but typical history associated with sweating and anxiety might be a pointer.

Her serum metanephrine were 265 pg/mL (normal <65 pg/mL). Her parathyroid hormone (PTH) levels were elevated 98 pg/mL (normal 10–55 pg/mL).

A CT scan showed a 5-cm mass **(Fig. 5)** at T11-L1 level in para-aortic area, and Iodine-131 metaiodobenzylguanidine (I0131 MIBG) scan confirmed a paraganglioma. After the resection of mass, the LV functions improved **(Videos 7 and 8)**.

Video 7 Video 8

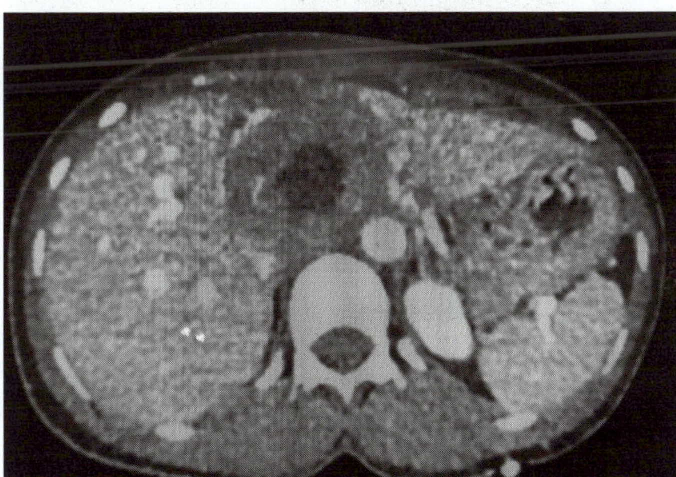

Fig. 5: Well-circumscribed peripherally enhancing mass of size 5 × 5.7 cm with central necrosis at the level of D11-L1 in aortocaval region.

Learning points: These two cases demonstrate that catecholamines excess can produce myocardial dysfunction (QT prolongation on ECG is seen in these cases, though it is not specific for it).

Further, these cases also highlight that clinical history is equally important in emergency or nonemergency situations.

Sidelights:

1. **Does Takotsubo cardiomyopathy occur on the right ventricle?**
2. **What does iPTH (intact parathyroid hormone) elevation in a paraganglioma suggest?**
3. **Revise the causes of ST elevation without MI.**

(*Sidelights are food for thought—provided to increase your curiosity:* So as a rule, do not read these answers before you try to answer them yourself. The answers provided here are not intended to be exhaustive).

Answer: Isolated right ventricular (RV) Takotsubo cardiomyopathy is rarely reported. There is reverse McConell sign in them (poor apical contractility and preserved basal contractility as opposed to what seen in pulmonary embolism, though not specific or sensitive sign.)

- Elevated iPTH in paraganglioma patient might suggest MEN [multiple endocrine neoplasia—(MEN 2/3)], sometimes even pheochromocytoma has high PTH secreted by the tumor.
- ST elevation may occur in the absence of myocardial infarction (MI) in Prinzmetal angina, pericarditis, Takotsubo cardiomyopathy, myopericarditis, early repolarization syndrome, in athletes, LV hypertrophy, left bundle branch block, Brugada syndrome, in patients with persistent LV aneurysm, as a reciprocal change to ST depression, in hyperkalemia, hypo and hypercalcemia, pulmonary embolism, subarachnoid hemorrhage, rarely in pneumothorax, pancreatitis, hiatus hernia, pheochromocytoma, hypothermia, cardiac metastasis, drugs like flecainide, and postcardioversion. Sometimes, artifact or ECG machine malfunction might be responsible! Spiked helmet sign on ECG in intensive care unit with severe critical illness is a new entity in the list of MI mimics.

CASE

10

Syncope or Seizure in a 50-year-old

"The whole is greater than the sum of the parts."

—Aristotle

A 50-year-old diabetic, hypertensive patient was brought to the emergency after an episode of loss of consciousness at home. He had two similar episodes in the last one and half months for which he was investigated and treated with levetiracetam. A brain MRI and an EEG were reportedly normal. All the episodes were very sudden, lasting a few minutes, associated with up rolling of eyeballs, and in one of the episode urinary incontinence was observed. In the last episode, the patient fell in the bathroom and had to be extricated by dismantling the door. However, the patient did not report any headaches, or amnesia on recovery in any of the episodes. He was taken to a local nursing home where an ECG was done **(Fig. 1)** and was subsequently referred to a tertiary care. The patient was hemodynamically stable, had clear consciousness, and did not complaint of any chest pain, or palpitation prior to the episode. His ECG at presentation at the referral center is shown in **Figure 2**. The troponins were not elevated (5.5 pg/mL) (normal <34 pg/mL). Creatine phosphokinase-MB (CPK-MB) was 97 U/L (normal <25 U/L). The other routine tests were unrevealing. An echocardiogram was suggestive of mild left ventricular (LV) apical hypokinesia with overall normal LV function.

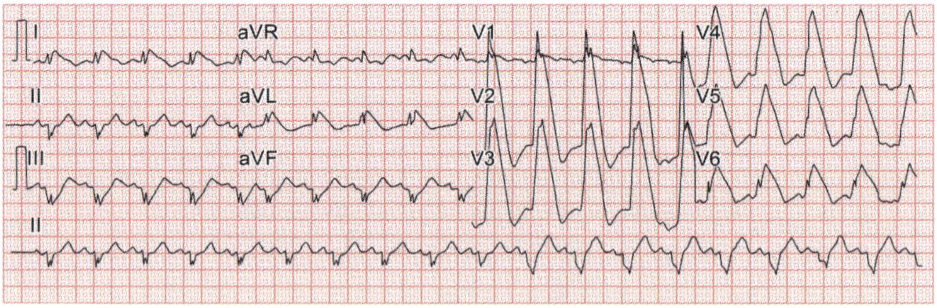

Fig. 1: The ECG done at a local facility after the event.

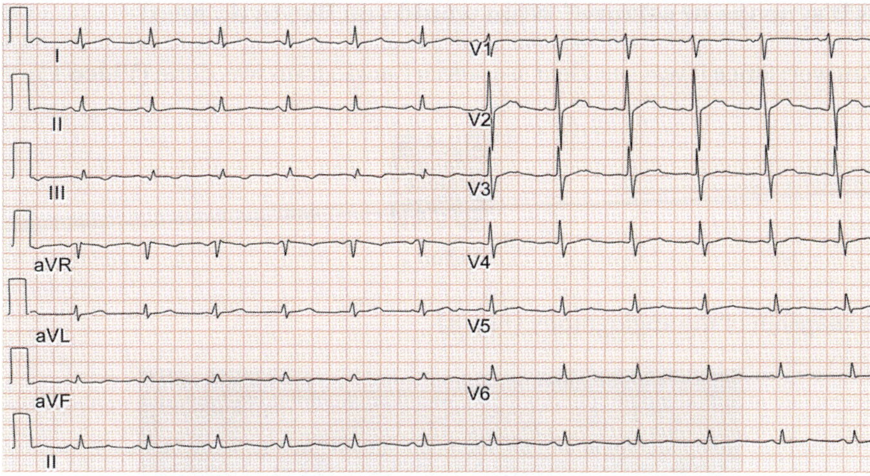

Fig. 2: The ECG on admission.

Is it syncope or seizure? What would you like to do next?

Answer: Since it was not clear, a coronary angiogram was done **(Video 1)**.

Video 1

A snapshot of the angiography **(Fig. 3)**

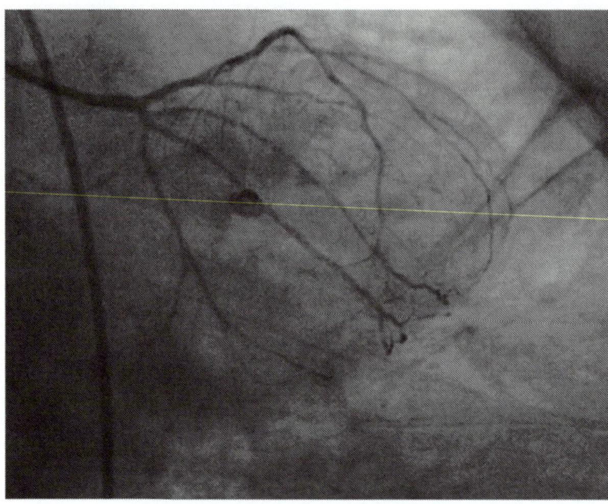

Fig. 3: Left coronary angiogram.

The angio showed no reflux and a left main coronary artery (LMCA) lesion was suspected. Because of the logistic reasons, the patient was planned for LMCA ostial angioplasty next day with ultrasound guidance.

How would you plan the procedure?

The next day angio are shown below—coronary injection in **Video 3** was done after that in **Video 2**.

Video 2 **Video 3**

What is the diagnosis?

Pause and think before you click the answer:

Answer: The patient developed severe chest pain and hypotension on wiring the left coronary artery. The ECG showed ST-segment elevations similar to Figure 1. On intracoronary nitroglycerine injection, the spasm was relieved with restoring the hemodynamics (Video 3). An intravascular ultrasound (IVUS) study was done that did not show any coronary ostial narrowing. Thus, the patient had coronary artery spasm responsible for the loss of consciousness events. Retrospectively, the patient IgE levels were 503 IU/mL (normal <100 IU/mL) and a history of frequent episodes of skin rashes requiring antiallergic medicines. The initial angiogram was also showing left main coronary spasm that was interpreted as ostial lesion; and also the coronary vessels were all mildly constricted that was not appreciated. His tryptase levels were mildly elevated. Thus the patient had a Kounis syndrome.

Learning points: Coronary artery spasm can cause syncope mimicking a seizure disorder.

Sidelights:

1. **When can syncope cause seizure, and seizure cause a syncope?**
2. **Can a patient on head-up tilt test (HuTT) develop syncope without bradycardia or hypotension?**

(*Sidelights are food for thought—provided to increase your curiosity:* So as a rule, do not read these answers before you try to answer them yourself. The answers provided here are not intended to be exhaustive.)

Answer: A prolonged syncope, especially if the patient is prevented from becoming horizontal, can lead to a few myoclonic jerks. Thus, malignant vasovagal syncope can provoke a seizure. More than 20 jerks would indicate seizure. During the tonic posturing or myoclonic jerks of syncope, there is no epileptic EEG. Temporal lobe seizures or seizures that spread to involve autonomic cortex areas might cause syncope due to ictal asystole or severe bradycardia. Not understanding this fact, permanent pacemaker has been implanted in seizure patients with no relief or recurrence of symptoms. Thus, a detailed analysis of history is needed to understand the cause of loss of consciousness.

- The common feeling is to diagnose a psychogenic or conversion reaction in this setting. But a rarely recognized syncope, hyperventilation syncope can occur in the absence of hypotension and significant bradycardia, due to hyperventilation induced drop in pCO_2 and cerebral vasoconstriction causing a genuine syncope!

CASE

11

PDA and PAH

"Haste denies all acts their dignity."

—Dante Alighieri

A 24-year-old lady presented with exertional breathlessness since childhood. She had a patent ductus arteriosus (PDA) with a systolic murmur and mild cardiomegaly. The cath data are as shown in the **Table 1**.

TABLE 1: Resting hemodynamic data.

		Basal
	mm Hg	*Sat%*
SVC	4	73
PA	117/76($\overline{92}$)	88
AO	160/82($\overline{110}$)	92
Qp/Qs	1.7:1	
PVRI (wood units.m^2)	13.3	

(AO: aorta; PA: pulmonary artery; PVRI: pulmonary vascular resistance index; Qp/Qs: pulmonary-to-systemic flow ratio; SVC: superior vena cava)

Her angiography is shown in **Video 1**.

Video 1

Should this PDA be closed? What are the considerations?

Pause and think before you click the answer:

Answer: This case teaches several important concepts. Her ECG and X-rays were not provided just for the sake of discussion. Ordinarily, a high pulmonary vascular resistance index (PVRI) (>6–8 U/m^2) in PDA would indicate inoperability. Also, a resting desaturation would contradict closure. But in an Eisenmenger PDA, one would not expect a 15% step up, some cardiomegaly and favorable ECG. The calculation of shunt in PDA is fraught with uncertainty as you cannot actually calculate shunt simply by averaging RPA and LPA saturation truly. Further, assumed VO_2 can be problematic as is well known. Hence, a particular number of PVRI should be viewed with caution. However, the basic dictum is "if in doubt, do not close the shunt". Since the patient condition after a "wrong decision" in these cases is much worse than that with a patent PDA with shunt reversal. The pressures in this case seem prohibitory. But difference in systolic pressures in aorta and PA is not like an inoperable PDA. With the total picture of a continuous murmur, left ventricular (LV) enlargement on echo, and systolic gradient with wide pulse pressure and good angiographic left-to-right shunt, a balloon occlusion of PDA was done. The resting saturation of 92% was unexpected and unexplained (in real-world scenario, we need to sometimes disregard a fact even though it is important, we do so if the hierarchy of reasoning suggests that it might be ok to do so). In this case, the balloon occlusion of PDA caused remarkable fall in PA pressures. Consequently, the ductus was closed with a large device **(Video 2)**. The post device closure, pressures were as follows **(Table 2)**.

Video 2

TABLE 2: Hemodynamic data immediately after closure.

After PDA device closure	
	mm Hg
RA	4
PA	40/14($\overline{25}$)
AO	162/72($\overline{106}$)
Qp/Qs	1
PVRI (wood units.m^2)	3

(AO: aorta; PA: pulmonary artery; PDA: patent ductus arteriosus; PVRI: pulmonary vascular resistance index; Qp/Qs: pulmonary-to-systemic flow ratio; RA: right atrium)

The balloon occlusion is best done with a short Fogarty balloon [PDA crossed from arterial side into pulmonary artery (PA) and then inflate balloon and withdraw to occlude the ductus], as longer balloons will obstruct the aorta or PA and might give erroneous results. An example of Fogarty occlusion in another patient is shown. In this case, a 6F Fogarty was not enough to close the duct (as seen in the **Video 3**) and a 7F Fogarty was used subsequently (not shown) (The PDA occlusion might be done with a device, but then the impulse to use the device might influence your decision or the device could be wasted).

Video 3

Thus, a comprehensive clinical assessment is always required for decisions regarding operability. The decision is much easier in another case shown below.

- A 12-year-old boy with PDA and pulmonary hypertension. His chest X-ray and cath data are shown below **(Fig. 1 and Table 3)**.

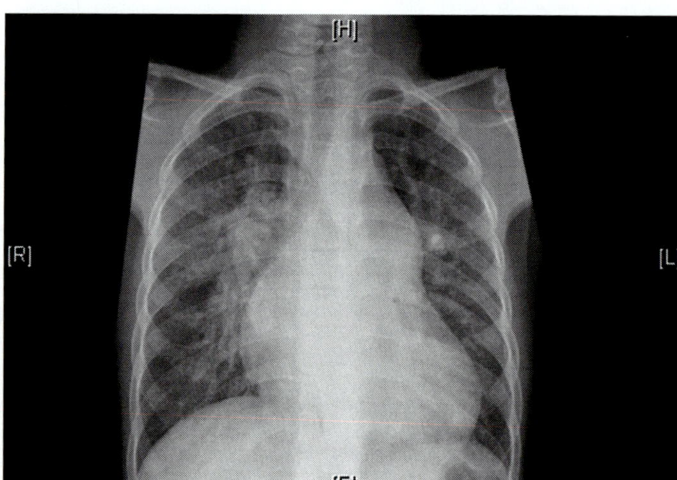

Fig. 1: Chest X-ray of 12-year-old boy with a PDA.

TABLE 3: Hemodynamic data.

		Basal
	mm Hg	***Sat%***
SVC	7	68
PA	107/67($\overline{86}$)	88
AO	134/70($\overline{92}$)	99
Qp/Qs	3:1	
PVRI (wood units.m^2)	10	

(AO: aorta; PA: pulmonary artery; PVRI: pulmonary vascular resistance index; Qp/Qs: pulmonary-to-systemic flow ratio; SVC: superior vena cava)

The angiogram showed a large duct with large shunt **(Video 4)**.

Video 4

The balloon occlusion tracings are shown in **Figures 2A and B**.

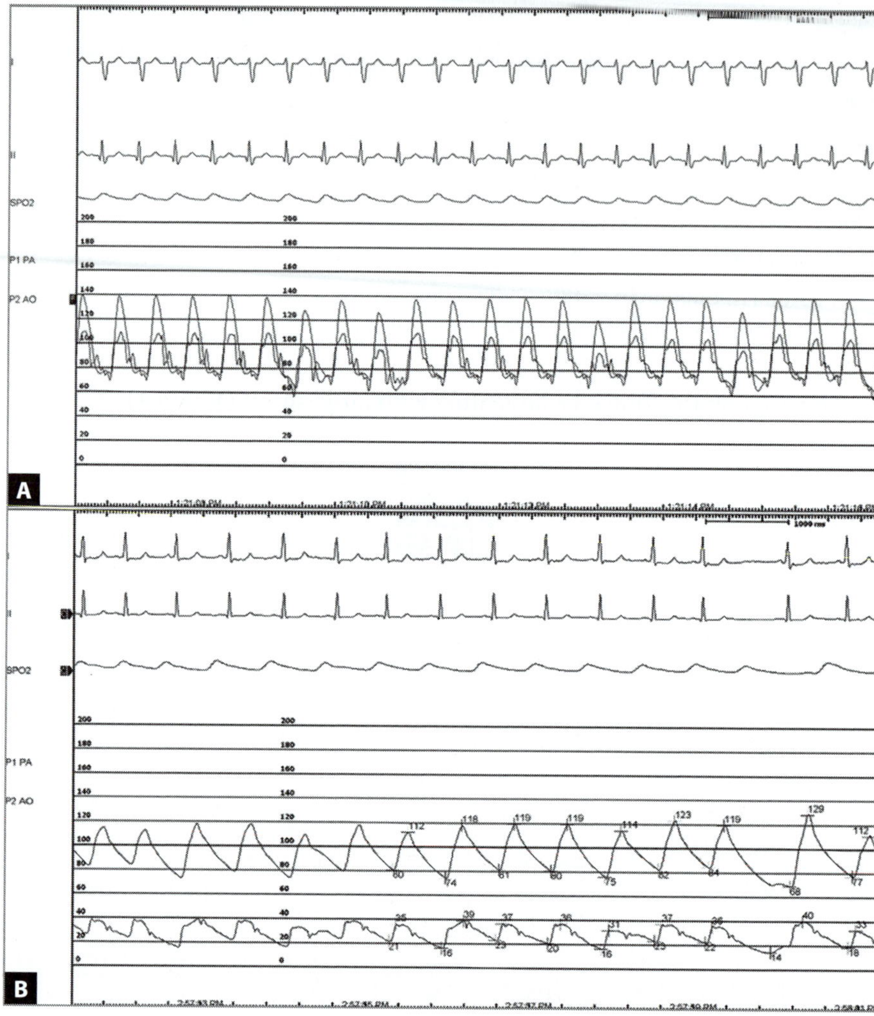

Figs. 2A and B: (A) Aortic and pulmonary artery (PA) pressure tracings before balloon occlusion of duct; (B) Postballoon occlusion.

TABLE 4: The hemodynamic data after the closure of the PDA.

After PDA device closure	
	mm Hg
RA	6
PA	34/17($\overline{27}$)
AO	110/62($\overline{85}$)
Qp/Qs	1
PVRI (wood units.m^2)	4

(AO: aorta; PA: pulmonary artery; PDA: patent ductus arteriosus; PVRI: pulmonary vascular resistance index; Qp/Qs: pulmonary-to-systemic flow ratio; RA: right atrium)

Caution: There should be significant fall in PA pressure with balloon occlusion if the PDA is to be closed with device or surgery. What constitutes a significant fall remains debatable, but one study showed that patients in whom the PA systolic pressure was more than half of aortic systolic pressure after the trial occlusion had persistent pulmonary arterial hypertension (PAH) on follow-up. (Zhang DZ, et al. Circ Cardiovasc Interv. 2014;7:473)

There are many more cases of harm done by adventurous closure with a device compared to benefit as seen in this case. The patients presented here are very unusual patients who have not developed pulmonary vascular disease in adulthood despite large ducts. Why some patients do not develop pulmonary vascular irreversible disease even with a large unrestrictive shunt is not understood. However, certainly they are the exceptions. Most often, a PDA with high PVRI in adults should not be closed. Usually, there will not be large or significant left-to-right shunt in those patients.

I do not believe that a treat, repair, and treat policy (i.e., giving pulmonary vasodilators and then closing the ductus) in them should be adopted.

The life of the patient with a closed PDA (if it was inoperable) could be far worse than life of a patient with ductus and Eisenmenger syndrome—a point that needs to be constantly remembered.

- An example of the child who had a device closure of PDA (with only slight fall in PA pressure) and presented with severe PAH and right ventricular (RV) failure 10 years later is shown below to impress upon you that "If in doubt, do not close" the PDA **(Figs. 3 and 4)**.

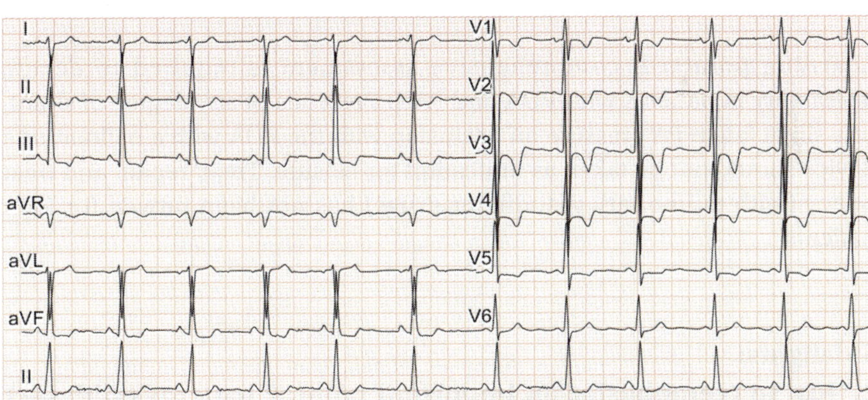

Fig. 3: ECG of a patient who had "wrongly" got patent ductus arteriosus closed.

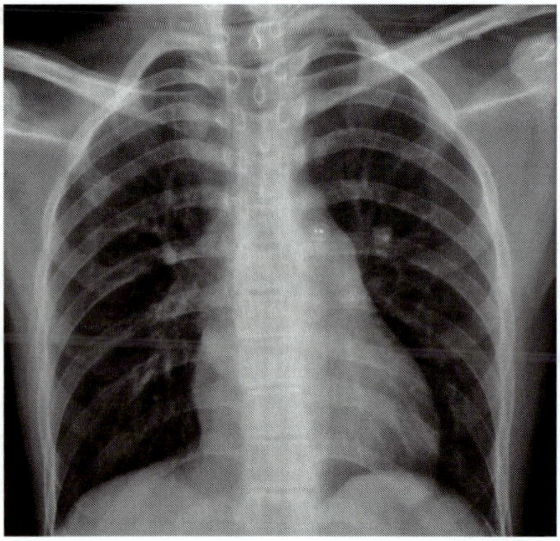

Fig. 4: Chest X-ray of the same patient showing device (*see* echo).

His PA pressure was nearly 100 mm Hg systolic and he was very symptomatic on triple therapy with pulmonary vasodilators **(Videos 5 and 6)**.

Video 5 **Video 6**

Learning points: A comprehensive assessment is required to decide operability in patients with PDA and PAH. Presence of any degree of shunt, or a slight fall in PA pressure on occlusion with the PDA with a balloon or a device should not be taken as indication for closure. Treat, repair, and treat policy (with pulmonary vasodilator drugs) has not been proven for PDA patients.

Sidelights:

1. **Just to reemphasize an important point, 2 patients (slides—1 and 2) with high PA pressures and its response to oxygen are shown. Which of the patients have VSD, and the other a PDA?**

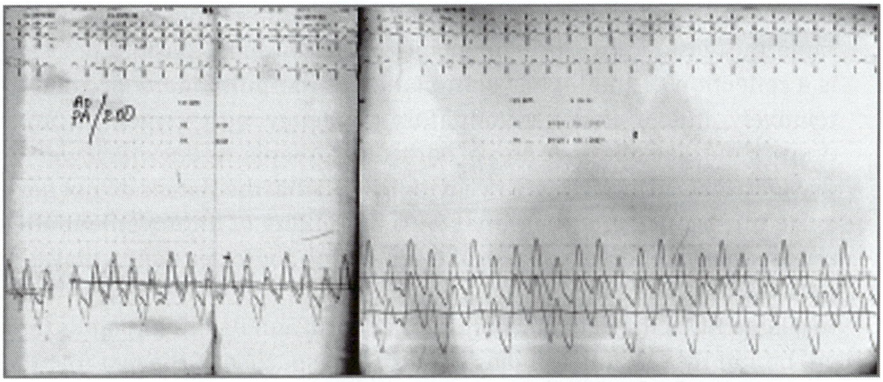

Slide 1: Aortic and pulmonary artery pressures resting (left), and after oxygen (right). (A very old slide.)

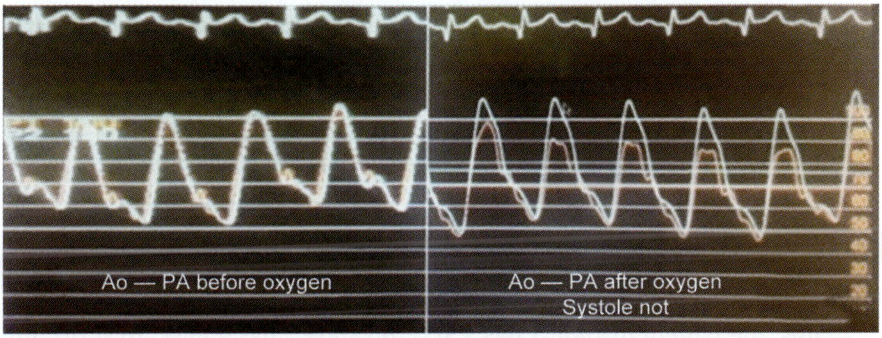

Slide 2: Aortic and pulmonary artery pressures resting (left), and after oxygen (right).

(*Slide courtesy:* Dr K Sivakumar)

2. Amongst the patients with Eisenmenger syndrome due to as atrial septal defect (ASD), VSD, or a PDA, which of the patients would have (A) heart failure, (B) hoarseness of voice, (C) wide pulse pressure more commonly (three different questions)?

(*Sidelights are food for thought—provided to increase your curiosity:* So as a rule, do not read these answers before you try to answer them yourself. The answers provided here are not intended to be exhaustive.)

Answer: In a patient with large unrestrictive VSD, the systolic pressures are same, the diastolic pressures might differ and a lower PA diastolic pressure is a reflection of the higher compliance of the pulmonary circulation relatively; thus if after a vasodilatory challenge with oxygen or other drugs, if the diastolic pressures of aorta and PA separate out with lower PA diastolic than aortic, it might be an indication that the vessels do not have a fixed resistance and there may be a possibility of improvement after operation. Of course, the wider the separation (or lower the PA diastolic pressure compared to aorta), the better it is.

In a large PDA, the diastolic pressures of aorta and PA are similar as they are bound by a channel in diastole also (irrespective of the fact that the shunt is left-to-right or right-to-left). With a large PDA shunt, the aortic pressures might be slightly higher than PA pressures as the LV volume of ejection is higher than RV. Thus a systolic separation in PDA is good news and the diastolic pressures lower the better (as aortic diastolic will be lower with a larger shunt as well as the PA diastolic will be lower as it has to be equal to the aortic pressure). Of course, this lower diastolic pressures might occur due to sever pulmonary regurgitation also that has to be factored into the decision. The patients with large shunt with lower diastolic pressure would have significant step up in PA, whereas the low diastolic because of the pulmonary regurgitation due to Eisenmenger syndrome would have no significant step up and would have systemic desaturation in lower limb.

Thus, the patient in slide 1 has VSD, and slide 2 has a PDA. In short, the dictum is diastolic separation in VSD indicate operability, and systolic separation in PDA indicates operability when you have aortic and PA tracings simultaneously.

- Amongst the patients of Eisenmenger syndrome, (A) heart failure is a late event in post-tricuspid shunt of VSD or PDA, but is not so rare in patients of ASD. The combined muscular power of both the right and left ventricle is operating in post-tricuspid shunt, whereas the right ventricle alone is facing the pressure load in ASD. (B) Hoarseness of voice is due to recurrent laryngeal nerve palsy from compression by a dilated PA or a hypertensive PDA and is more common with patients of PDA, and ASD Eisenmenger syndrome; (C) wide pulse pressure in Eisenmenger syndrome does not occur unless the patient of a PDA has pulmonary regurgitation. Wide pulse pressure does not occur in patients with ASD or VSD Eisenmenger unless they have another unrelated cause for it, but is not uncommon with PDA Eisenmenger syndrome.

CASE

12

PDA and PAH with Cyanosis

"There's no need for fiction in medicine, for the facts will always beat anything you fancy."

—Arthur Conan Doyle

An 8-year-old child presented with history of recurrent lower respiratory infections since infancy. He had developed increasing breathlessness for last 4 years. On examination, he had differential cyanosis with saturation in lower limbs at 66%. His chest X-ray is shown in **Figure 1**. ECG showed right axis deviation with right ventricular hypertrophy.

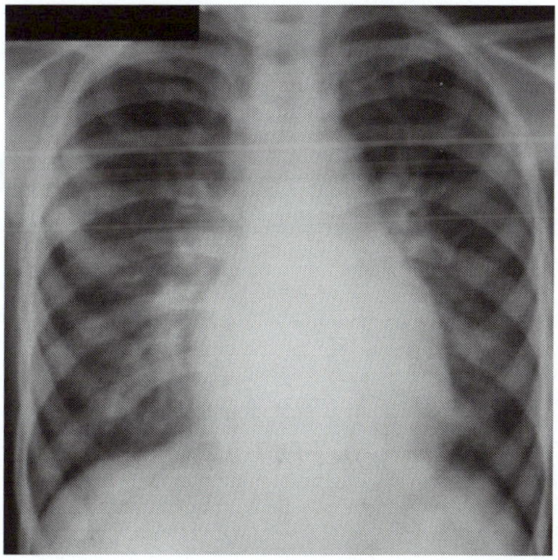

Fig. 1: Chest X-ray.

The left ventricular angiogram shows patent ductus arteriosus (PDA) with bidirectional shunt, mainly right-to-left shunting **(Video 1)**.

Video 1

The limited catheter data are shown in **Table 1**.

TABLE 1: Limited catheterization data.

	mm Hg	*Saturation %*
RA	7	58
RV	106/7–8	
PA	108/76($\overline{90}$)	62
AO	116/76($\overline{92}$)	96 (AO), **66 (FA)**
PVRI (wood units.m^2)	26 (19 on O_2)	

(AO: aorta; FA: femoral artery; PA: pulmonary artery; PVRI: pulmonary vascular resistance index; RA: right atrium; RV: right ventricle)

Can he be operated?

The child was operated. In addition to PDA closure, another cardiac procedure was done. Can you now guess what could that be?

Pause and think before you click the answer:

Answer: The complete catheterization data are shown in **Table 2**.

TABLE 2: Complete catheterization data.

	mm Hg	*Saturation %*
RA	7	58
RV	106/7–8	
PA	108/76($\overline{90}$)	62
AO	116/76($\overline{92}$)	66 **(FA)**
PVRI (wood units.m^2)	26 (19 on O_2)	
PAW	a 45 v 46($\overline{38}$)	92%
MVA	**0.5 cm^2**	

(AO: aorta; FA: femoral artery; MVA: mitral valve area; PA: pulmonary artery; PAW: pulmonary artery wedge PVRI: pulmonary vascular resistance index; RA: right atrium; RV: right ventricle)

Patient with PDA and differential cyanosis is inoperable. A pulmonary vascular resistance index (PVRI) of 29 wood units is prohibitively high. However, this patient underwent surgical treatment of PDA closure and in addition mitral valve repair for severe mitral stenosis. He had severe mitral stenosis (MVA—0.5 cm^2). The presence of mitral stenosis [postcapillary pulmonary hypertension (PH)] somehow protects from the irreversible pulmonary vascular changes. You must have seen suprasystemic pulmonary artery pressures becoming almost normal after balloon mitral valvuloplasty. Thus, this child had significant improvement, though the catheterization 2 years later, still had some pulmonary arterial hypertension (PAH), but he had normal effort tolerance and was in NYHA class 1. His PA pressures 2 years after operation are shown in **Figure 2**.

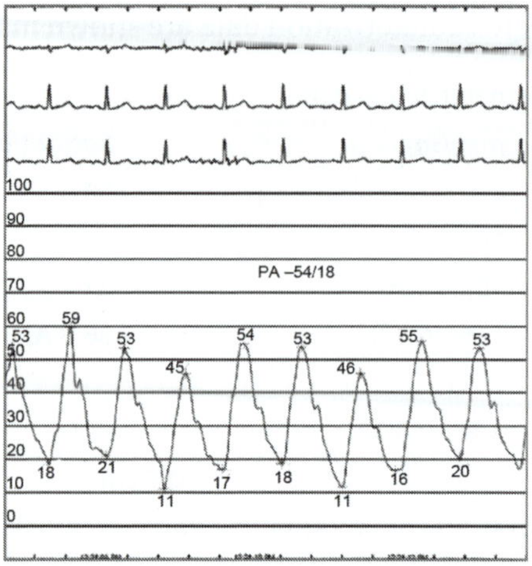

Fig. 2: Postoperative catheterization data after 2 years.

(*Source:* Gupta A, Kothari SS. Operable patent ductus arteriosus even with differential cyanosis: A case of patent ductus arteriosus and mitral stenosis. Cardiol Young. 2017;27(9):1845-8.)

Learning points: Differential cyanosis in PDA denotes severe PH and inoperability. But in presence of severe postcapillary PH, the raised PVRI may be substantially reversible. There are limited cases for decision making in this subset, but this point should be carefully considered. The raised PVRI in patients with postcapillary hypertension from mitral stenosis is mostly reversible, irrespective of the value of PVRI, if the mitral stenosis is treated. In some patients, the rise in postcapillary pressures generates a very significant reactive precapillary PAH, whereas in others this rise is not severe. The irreversible histological changes of plexiform lesions in the pulmonary vasculature are not seen in mitral stenosis patients.

Sidelights: What are the other causes of reversible PAH?

(*Sidelights are food for thought—provided to increase your curiosity:* So as a rule, do not read these answers before you try to answer them yourself. The answers provided here are not intended to be exhaustive.)

Answer: Typically PAH due to hypoxia, hypercarbia, and acidosis is reversible by treating the primary cause. When faced with a patient of PH, it is well to remember to optimize the physiological factors that might even partially reduce the PA pressure (and thus help the patients even with otherwise irreversible pulmonary hypertensive disorders like Eisenmenger syndrome.) Thus optimizing the hematocrit, blood volume, and lung volumes will help reduce the PA pressures accordingly.

Postcapillary PH may be ameliorated to a large extent if the disorder causing it is treated as shown in this case report. Mitral stenosis, cor triatriatum, and some forms of pulmonary venous stenosis may be fully treatable. If raised left ventricular end-diastolic pressure (LVEDP) is the problem causing PH, and the cause is partially or completely treated, it might improve the PA pressures. For example, treatment of aortic stenosis, hypertension, and constrictive pericarditis will reduce the PA pressures in patients with these disorders. A phenotype of heart failure with preserved ejection fraction might present with severe PAH and, though the current vasodilator therapy is not useful in these patients, PH may conceivably improve with the treatment of the primary disorder in the future.

The PAH due to high pulmonary blood flow from shunt lesions (hyperkinetic PH) is completely reversed by closure of the shunt before it has caused obstructive changes.

Obstruction in the pulmonary arteries by pulmonary thromboembolism (chronic thromboembolic PH), or PAH due to peripheral pulmonary arterial stenosis from a variety of causes may be treatable.

Pulmonary vasculitis, PH due to hypervolemia and other factors in kidney disease, PAH with hemolytic anemia may be partially reversible. Treatment of any cause of anemia (by reducing the hypervolemia or cardiac output) or polycythemia (by decreasing the viscosity) helps to optimize the PA pressures. Similarly, the optimizing of lung volumes avoiding collapse or hyperinflation reduces the PH.

Airway obstruction from compression by pulmonary arteries or other vessels such as vascular rings, upper airway obstruction from adenoids or other structures, and obstructive sleep apnea are other important causes of treatable PH. Rarely, infants with beriberi may masquerade as PH. Finally, portopulmonary hypertension and Abernethy syndrome (extrahepatic portosystemic shunt) as a cause of treatable PH must not be overlooked.

CASE

13

Another PAH and Cyanosis

"Wonder is the beginning of wisdom."

—**Socrates**

A 25-year-old lady presented with severe cyanosis and dyspnea since early childhood. Her evaluation showed a small atrial septal defect (ASD) with right-to-left shunt and severe pulmonary arterial hypertension (PAH). Her resting oxygen saturation was 85%. The chest X-ray is shown in **Figure 1**. The ECG showed right axis deviation and severe right ventricular hypertrophy (RVH). On cardiac catheterization, the pulmonary artery (PA) pressures were markedly elevated at 120/70 (mean 95 mm Hg) in the main PA and in the left PA (aortic pressure 110/70 mm Hg). However, the right PA could not be entered. Instead, it arose from the aorta. An aortogram showed the origin of right pulmonary artery (RPA) but was atretic soon after **(Fig. 2)**. The distal part of reformed RPA was seen in the CT angiogram **(Figs. 3A to C)**.

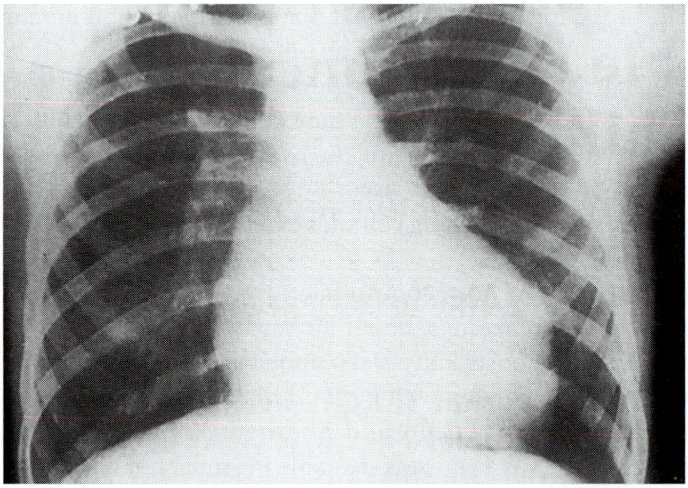

Fig. 1: Chest X-ray.

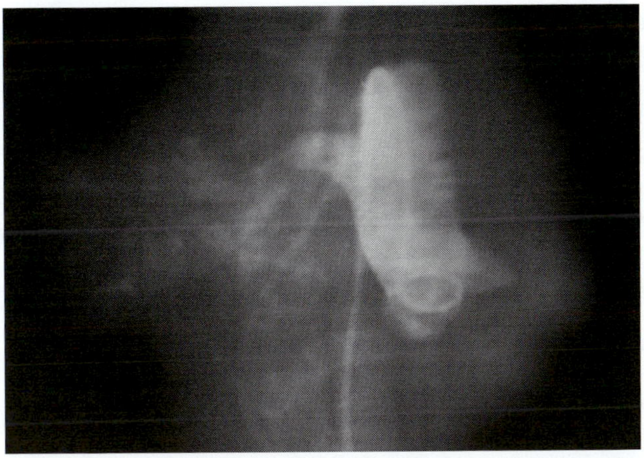

Fig. 2: Aortogram shows atretic right pulmonary artery arising from ascending aorta.

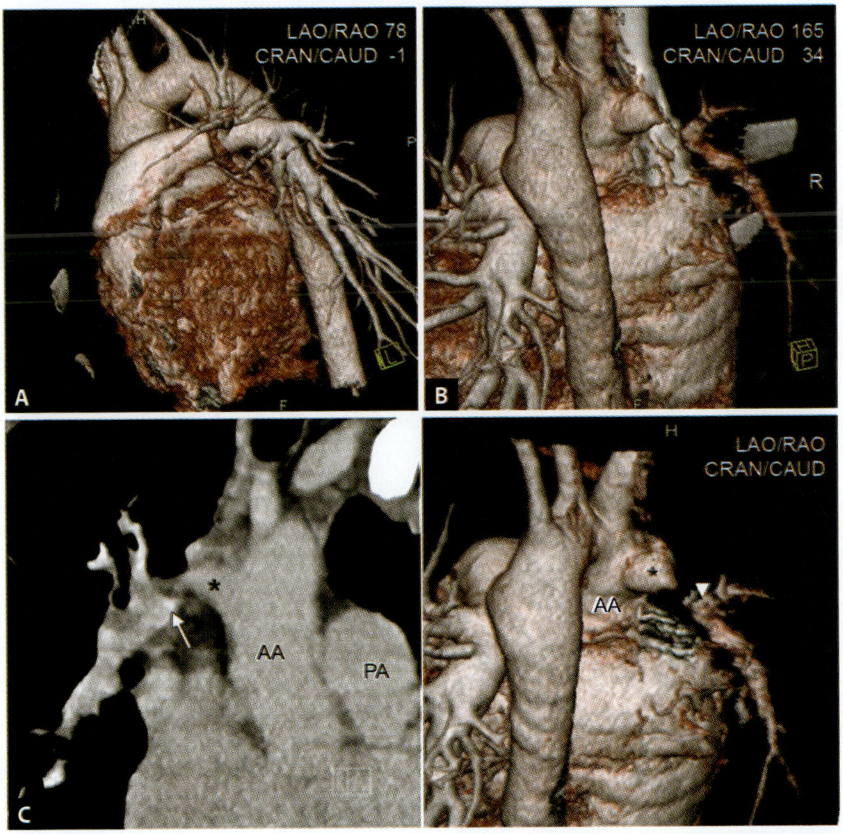

Figs. 3A to C: (A) Volume-rendered CT image shows MPA continuing as LPA. A ductal ampulla is also seen; (B) Posterior view shows distal RPA reformed. The RPA is arising from ascending aorta but is atretic soon after origin; and (C) The anatomy in anterior and posterior aspect (arrows show distal RPA). (AA; ascending aorta; PA: pulmonary artery; LPA: left pulmonary artery; MPA: main pulmonary artery; RPA: right pulmonary artery)

Can anything be done to improve her symptoms?

Pause and think before you click the answer:

Answer: When one PA arises from the aorta that particular lung receives aortic pressure in the lung and develops changes of pulmonary vascular disease. The other lung which receives the entire blood flow from the systemic venous return also develops vascular disease as it is receiving high pulmonary blood flow. Therefore, the operative management of hemitruncus (i.e., one PA arising from aorta) requires early correction in infancy. The situation in this patient is different because of severe ostial stenosis/atresia at origin; hence the right lung was "protected". The right and the left pulmonary arteries are like two circuits in parallel. The mean resistance of total lung (R) is denoted by the formula:

$1/R = 1/R1 + 1/R2$ (where R1 and R2 are resistances in right and left lung respectively).

Hence, it follows that R will always be lower than the lower value of R1 or R2. Thus, if either of the lung is having a normal pulmonary vascular resistance index (PVRI), the resultant lung resistance would be normal if the two lungs could be connected, theoretically at least. For example, if the PVRI in left lung is 20 units and that in the right lung is 5 units, the mean resistance after joining the 2 will be (<5) 3.33 units. Although, the exact resistance in right lung was not known, the two arteries were connected by a Dacron graft **(Video 1)** and after that the mean PA pressure fell to 57 mm Hg. The patient's saturation markedly improved. On follow-up after 2 years, she was in NYHA class 1. Longer follow-up would be desirable but she was lost to follow up (just recanalizing the RPA and placing a covered stent in the RPA would not change the PA pressures and the right lung would be Eisenmengerized in due course, hence that approach was not taken, although it appeared tempting to do so by just looking at the anatomy).

Video 1

This case highlights the complexity in the of management of patients with disconnected PAs, and provides a framework for theoretic reasoning. The exact quantification of PVRI is now possible with the help of MRI, as MRI can give the regional pulmonary blood flow (pressures obtained from cardiac catheterization and flows across each PA obtained from MRI, regional PVRI can be calculated).

(*Source:* Talwar S, Kothari SS, Sharma P, Chauhan S, Gulati GS, Choudhary SK, et al. Successful surgical correction of anomalous origin of the right pulmonary artery from the aorta in an adult. J Card Surg. 2011;26(2):201-4.)

Learning points: The pulmonary vascular resistance (R) can be thought of as 1/R = 1/R1 + 1/R2, R1, and R2 are resistances in right and left pulmonary arteries. Thus, as long as one lung is having low PVRI, the patient may be operable (that is why one lung transplantation was also effective in Eisenmenger syndrome, although now a days bilateral lung transplant is common).

Sidelights:

1. **What is the PA pressure after a pneumonectomy of one lung in adults?**
2. **What is the PA pressures in the main PA in infants with absent one PA?**
3. **What is the PA pressure in patients with partial anomalous pulmonary venous connections (PAPVC)?**

(*Sidelights are food for thought—provided to increase your curiosity:* So as a rule, do not read these answers before you try to answer them yourself. The answers provided here are not intended to be exhaustive.)

Answer: The PA pressure does not significantly change after pneumonectomy (as was done for tuberculosis of one lung in the past), and this is to emphasize that the pulmonary disorder to cause PAH must be extensive: Thus in chronic obstructive pulmonary disease (COPD) only mild PAH is seen. Or mild PAH in lung disease indicates severe pulmonary disease. A mean PA pressure of 35 mm Hg is considered severe PAH for lung disorders. If lung disease is causing severe hypoxia, then significant PAH might ensue.

- Contrary to the situation described above, if there is only 1 PA from infancy, significant PAH is the rule in that normally supplied lung also, even though the lung is receiving only twice the pulmonary blood flow as compared to normal infants with two pulmonary arteries, and lungs can accommodate a lot of blood flow as seen in patients after pneumonectomy! The abnormal lung receiving the PA from aorta of course can get Eisenmengerized with high flow as expected (the patient described above had stenosis at origin of the anomalous PA and that protected the lung from high-flow vascular changes). Perhaps, there are fetal developmental alterations at play in hemitruncus. But if the hemitruncus is operated early in infancy, normalization of PAH is the rule.
- Partial anomalous pulmonary vein generally does not cause a large shunt and PA pressures are mildly elevated unless the pulmonary vein is obstructed. But in infants with scimitar syndrome, one often (not always) see severe PAH without pulmonary venous obstruction. Treatment of the aortopulmonary collaterals associated with scimitar syndrome does not reduce the PA pressure much. Perhaps, the vasculature in the lung is developmentally abnormal in some of the infants with scimitar syndrome.

CASE

14

PAH and Heart Failure

"When you don't cover up the world with words and labels, a sense of the miraculous returns to your life that was lost a long time ago when humanity, instead of using thought, became possessed by thought."

—Eckhart Tolle

A 12-year-old child had exertional breathlessness for last 5 years and had developed mild pedal edema for last 1 year. His chest X-ray is shown in **Figure 1**. It is apparent that he has marked cardiomegaly, the patient was in gross congestive heart failure with the jugular venous pressure (JVP) markedly elevated.

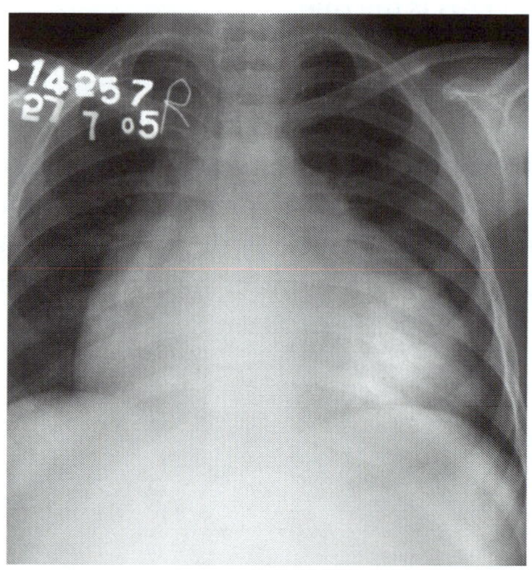

Fig. 1: Chest X-ray showing marked cardiomegaly.

The ECG showed severe right ventricular hypertrophy. The echo showed severe pulmonary arterial hypertension (PAH) with moderate tricuspid regurgitation (TR) and predicted right ventricular systolic pressure (RVSP) of 90 mm Hg. He was diagnosed as idiopathic PAH. The left heart was normal. He was taken for a cardiac catheterization. The right atrial pressure was 18 mm Hg. The systolic pressure in right ventricle and the main pulmonary artery (PA) was as 80 mm Hg. But something was missed, and after an intervention in the catheterization lab, the PA pressure was reduced.

What could that be?

Pause and think before you click the answer:

Answer: The PA angiogram unexpectedly revealed bilateral peripheral PA stenosis that was missed on clinical examination **(Fig. 2)**. A murmur in the chest in patients with pulmonary artery stenosis (PAS) is not uncommon, but might not be heard in all cases or in severe peripheral PS. This patient underwent balloon dilatation of peripheral PAS with significant clinical improvement **(Fig. 3)** (he was planned for staged intervention of the other side).

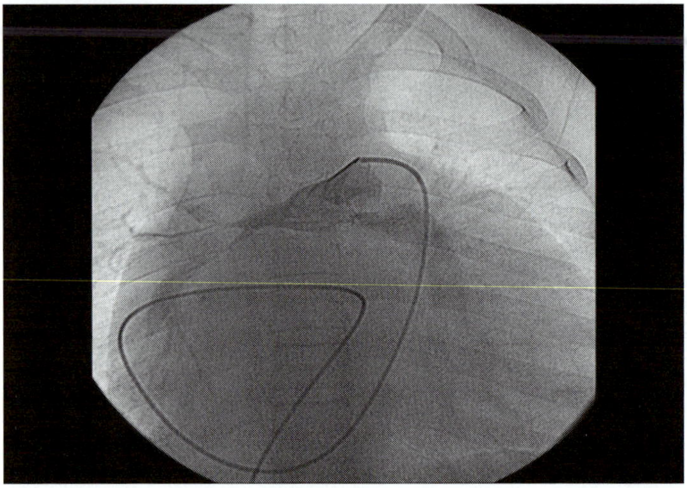

Fig. 2: Pulmonary artery (PA) angiogram shows severe bilateral pulmonary artery stenosis (PAS).

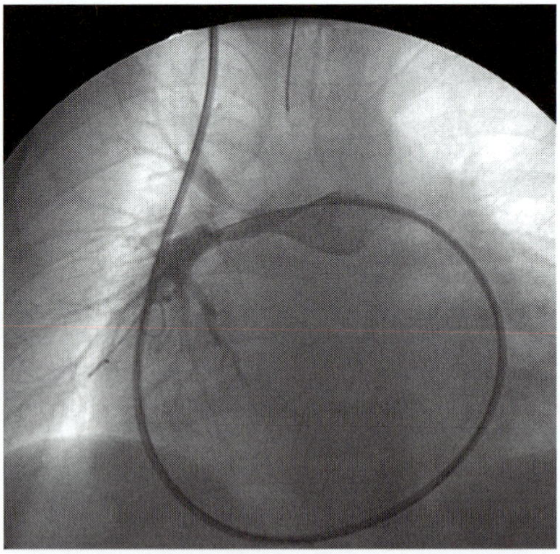

Fig. 3: Balloon dilatation of the right pulmonary artery (RPA) resulted in modest angiographic but significant clinical improvement. Now a days, this could be treated with stent implantation.

The X-ray, in retrospect, was showing pulmonary oligemia and that could have alerted to the possibility of peripheral PS. But gross cardiomegaly covering the lung fields might make the assessment difficult sometimes. Peripheral oligemia might also be seen in "real" severe PAH patients. See the similar X-ray of another patient with PAH and no peripheral PS **(Fig. 4)**. One can see the dilated PA through the cardiac silhouette in this patient with real PAH even as the peripheral lung fields seem oligemic.

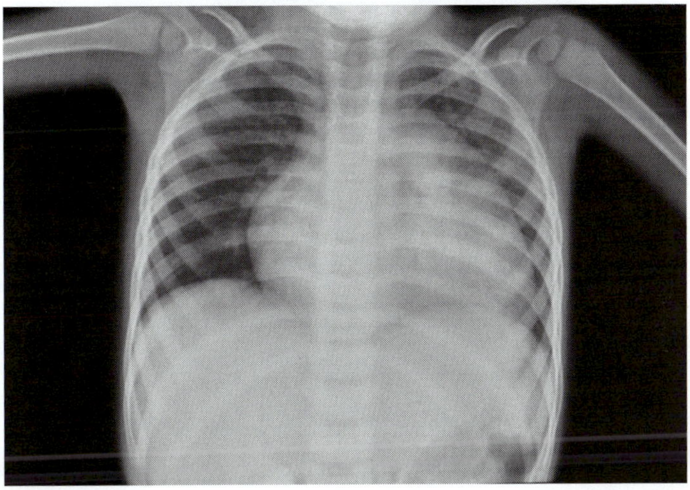

Fig. 4: Chest X-ray of a patient with severe pulmonary arterial hypertension (PAH) showing peripheral oligemia.

The representative CT frames of this patient shows the dilated PAs that were hidden within the cardiac silhouette **(Figs. 5A and B)**.

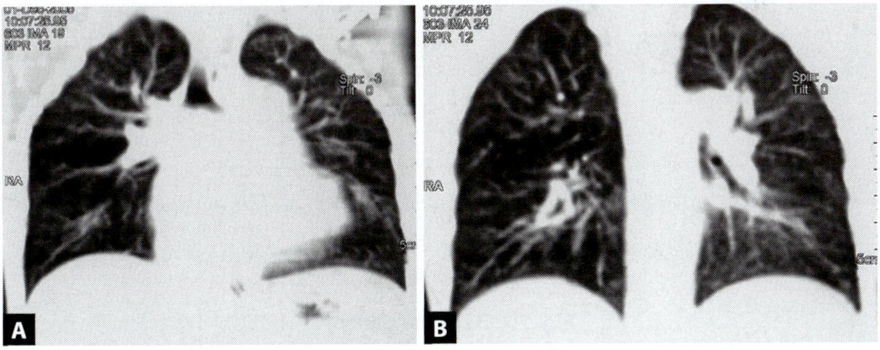

Figs. 5A and B: CT frames showing dilated RPA and LPA (sections at different levels to show RPA and LPA). (LPA: left pulmonary artery; RPA: right pulmonary artery)

But one may not be thinking right all the time and it is important for the clinician to try and think right all the time! More of it further on.

- A 10 year-old girl presented with exertional breathlessness on ordinary activity and anasarca for the last 6 months. She had intermittent fever and malaise for 1 year also. Her clinical examination suggested severe TR and pulmonary hypertension. Her chest X-ray **(Fig. 6)** and ECG **(Fig. 7)** are shown below. The inflammatory markers were mildly elevated, tests for systemic autoimmune diseases were negative.

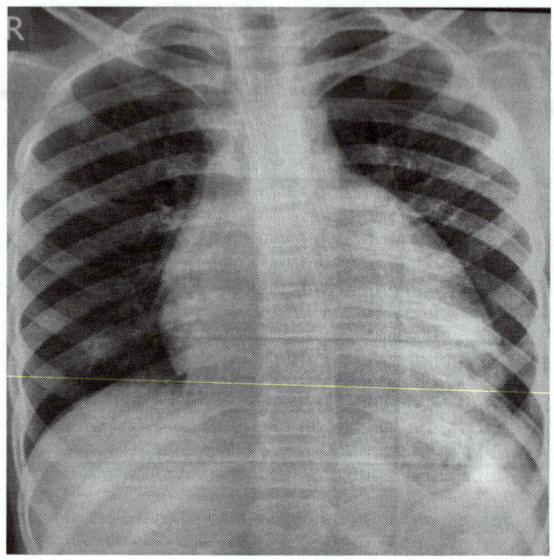

Fig. 6: Chest X-ray.

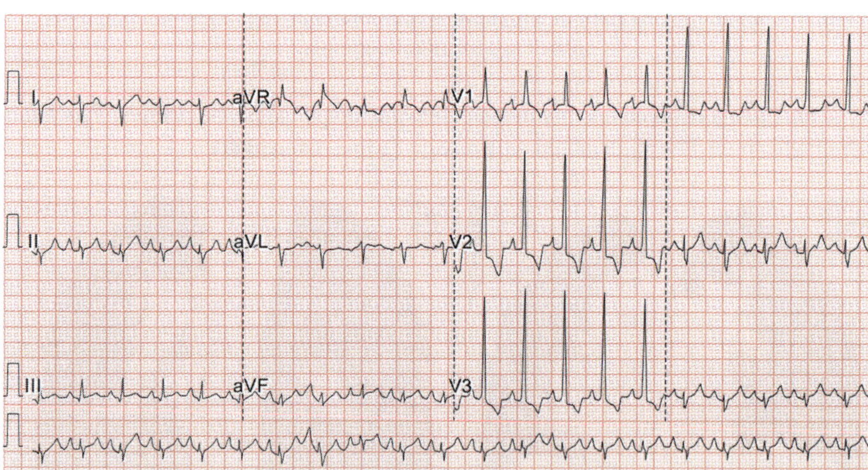

Fig. 7: ECG of the patient.

The echo showed severe hypertensive TR **(Fig. 8)**.

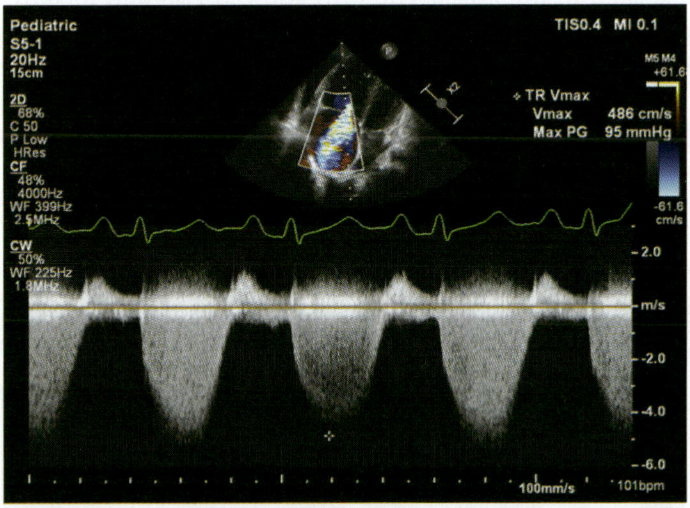

Fig. 8: Echo showing severe TR.

This time we could appreciate narrowing in the proximal pulmonary arteries on echocardiogram, and hence a CT was done **(Fig. 9)**. The patient had no syndromes known to be associated with congenital peripheral PAS, nor any significant family history of cardiac disease. All the peripheral pulses were normal and symmetrical.

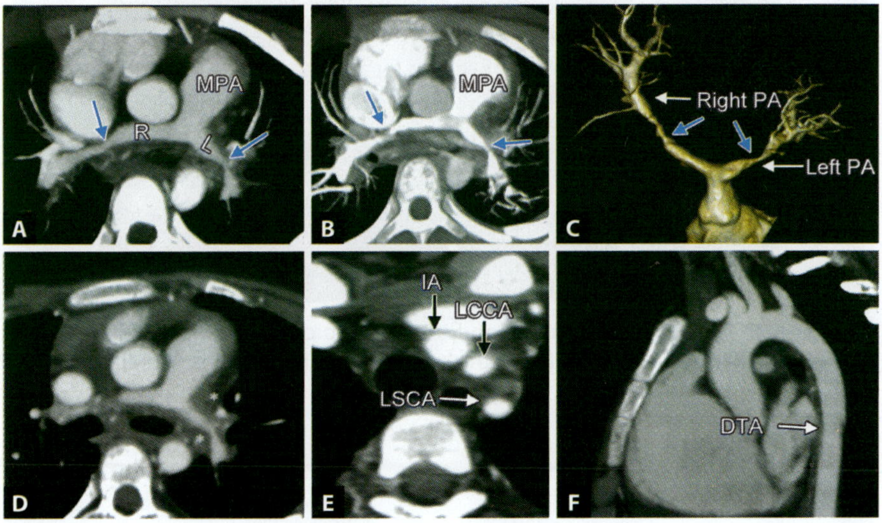

Fig. 9: The CT scan images. (DTA: descending thoracic aorta; IA: innominate artery; LCCA: left common carotid artery; LSCA: left subclavian artery. *Note:* *Denotes ill-defined soft tissue around pulmonary arteries.)

Although Takayasu aortoarteritis causing PAS is recognized, there was no disease seen in the aorta. The MRI showed PAS and focal thickening in the pulmonary arterial vessel wall **(Figs. 10A to D)**. A fluorine-18 fluorodeoxyglucose positron emission tomography (FDG PET) further confirmed the presence of inflammation in the lungs in the area of interest **(Fig. 11)**.

After comprehensive evaluation, she was diagnosed to have Takayasu arteritis causing pulmonary arterial stenosis. She was treated with steroids and palliative balloon dilatation of both the pulmonary arteries. She had flare of the disease on steroid withdrawal and needed longer term steroids and immunosuppression as well. This is quite a rare patient having PAS from inflammatory arteritis and with no apparent involvement of aorta yet.

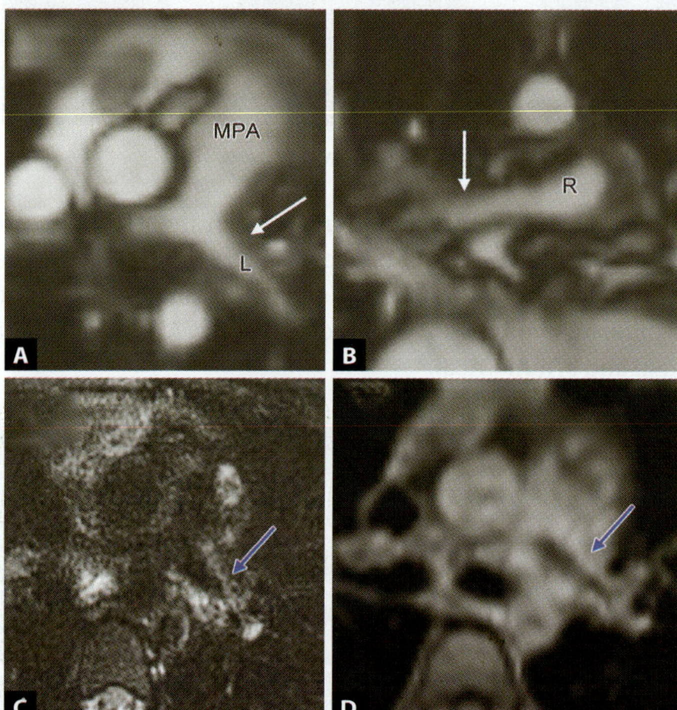

Figs. 10A to D: (A and B) Bright blood images depicting mural thickening along pulmonary arteries (arrows). (C) Mural thickening shows hyperintensity on fat saturated T2 image and (D) enhancement on postcontrast image. (MPA: main pulmonary artery; R: right pulmonary artery.)

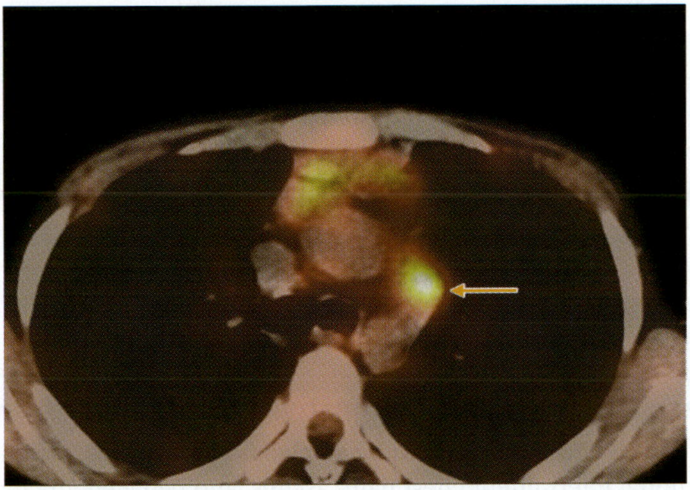

Fig. 11: Focal areas of Increased FDG uptake on fused PET CT along the Pulmonary artery. (FDG: fluorine-18 fluorodeoxyglucose; PET: positron emission tomography) (*Source:* Karuru UD, Relan J, Verma M, Kumar S, Tripathi M, Gupta SK, et al. Heart Failure in a Child: Multimodality Approach Leading to an Unusual Cause. JACC Case Rep. 2021;3(17):1869-76).

Learning point: Remember to exclude peripheral PAS in patients of PAH.

Sidelights: Can you enumerate all the causes of PAS?

(*Sidelights are food for thought—provided to increase your curiosity:* So as a rule, do not read these answers before you try to answer them yourself. The answers provided here are not intended to be exhaustive.)

Answer: Pulmonary artery stenosis is a part of William–Beuren syndrome, Alagille syndrome, Noonan syndrome, and congenital rubella syndrome. It often occurs in cyanotic congenital heart defects such as tetralogy of Fallot and similar diseases. Acquired PA stenosis is known in Chronic Thromboembolic Pulmonary Hypertension (CTEPH), Takayasu aortitis, sarcoidosis, histoplasmosis, fibrosing mediastinitis, IGG4-related disease, and from tumors, etc.

Now that you have mastered peripheral PS, read the following similar yet different case.

Case 14A: PAH and Congestive Heart Failure Again

A 6-year-old child was admitted with complaints of progressive breathlessness, nonexertional intermittent chest pain, ascites, and pedal edema for the last 4 months. There were no significant complaints in infancy or earlier years. Her growth and development had been normal and she did not appear "syndromic". She had jaundice 4 months ago, and was treated as viral hepatitis then. Her symptoms rapidly worsened over 3–4 months and she was in gross congestive heart failure. She had severe TR and PAH on echo. Her chest X-ray is shown in **Figure 12**.

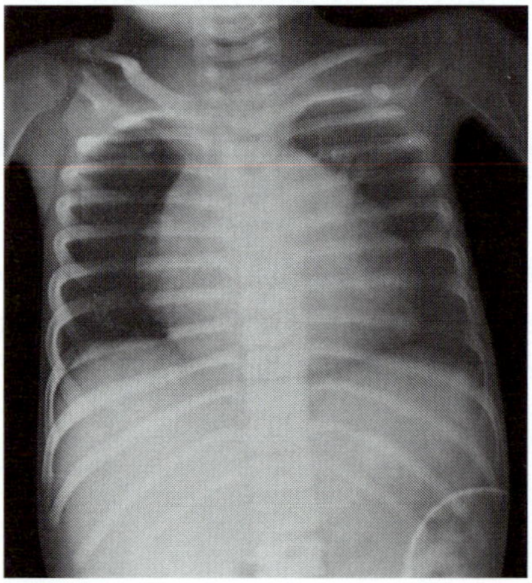

Fig. 12: Chest X-ray PA view showing cardiomegaly, right atrium and right ventricular enlargement, right ventricular type of apex, oligemic lung fields, and prominent bands to left upper lobe.

The echo **(Fig. 13 and Video 1)** showed severe TR, right ventricular dilatation and dysfunction, and dilated right atrium with a thrombus.

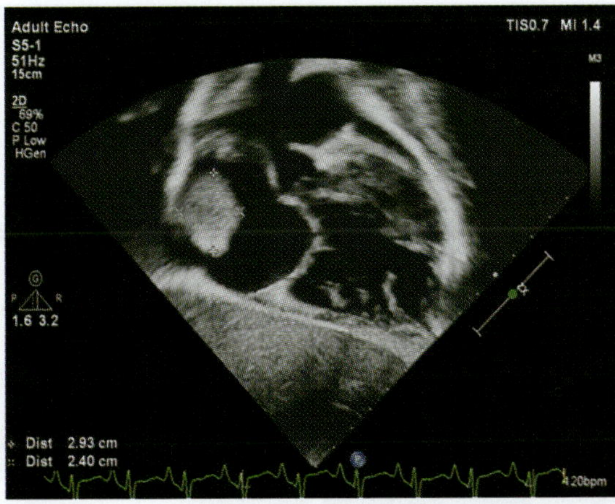

Fig. 13: Echo showing dilated right ventricle (RV) and a right atrium (RA) thrombus.

Video 1

The contrast-enhanced CT showed multiple lymph nodes, doubtful soft tissue mass surrounding the PAs, and abrupt cutoff of RPA **(Figs. 14A to D)**. The FDG-PET showed enhancement in the lymph nodes as shown in **Figures 15A to H**.

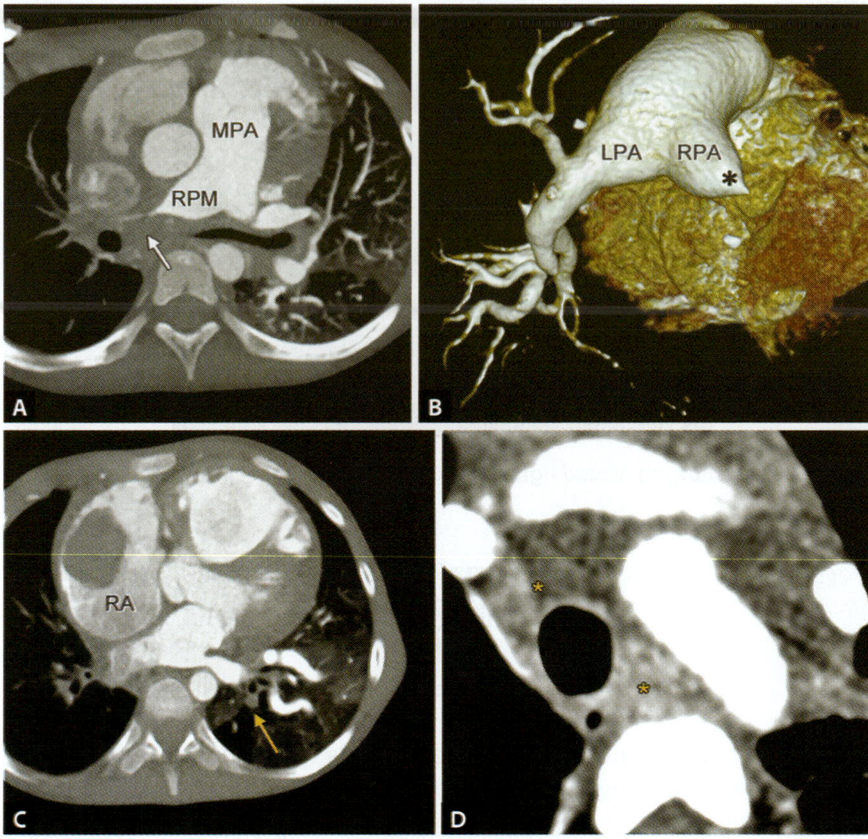

Figs. 14A to D: (A and B) CT angiography axial image depicting enlarged main pulmonary artery (MPA) with diffuse significant post-ostial stenosis of right pulmonary artery (RPA) (marked with white arrow). Volume rendered image from posterior view depicting abrupt cut off of RPA (white asterisk) and diminished flow on right side. Axial image depicting (C) dilated right atrium (RA) with thrombus and filling defect in one of sub-segmental branch of left descending PA (marked with yellow arrow). Mediastinal window (D) depicting multiple enlarged peripherally enhancing lymph nodes in pre-tracheal region (yellow asterisk). (*Figure reproduced with permission from:* J Am Coll Cardiol Case Reports. 2024;29(19):102569.)

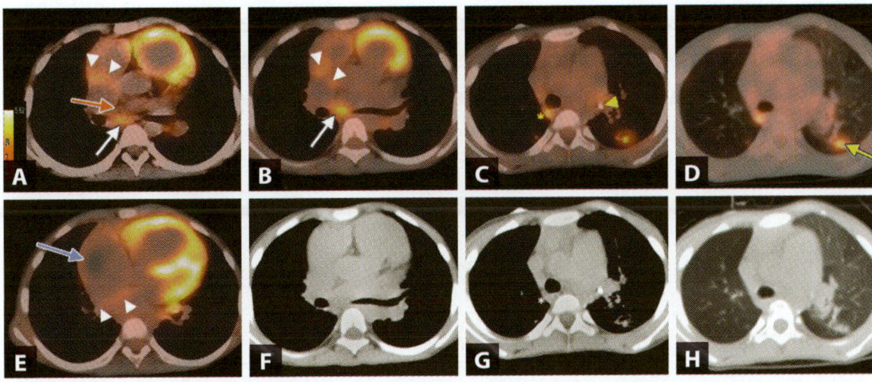

Figs. 15A to H: Axial sections of fused fluorine-18 fluorodeoxyglucose positron emission tomography/computed tomography (18F-FDG PET/CT) (A and E) corresponding to CT angiography (A and C) reveals increased FDG (white arrow) uptake posterior to the narrowed segment of right PA (red arrow) corresponding to soft tissue density lesion (likely lymph nodes) extending up to the sub-carinal region superiorly as seen in fused PET/CT (B) and corresponding non contrast CT (C). Ill defining thickening with increased FDG uptake is seen in the middle mediastinum along the RA and large vessels (A, B, and E—white arrow heads). Photopenic area seen in right atrium (E—blue arrow) corresponds to the thrombus in CT angiography (C). Increased FDG uptake in right ventricle is seen in addition to physiological uptake in left ventricle (A, B, and E) is likely secondary to pulmonary hypertension. Increased FDG uptake noted in the paratracheal lymph nodes (C and G—yellow asterisk) with non-FDG avid calcified left hilar lymph nodes (C and G—yellow arrowhead). FDG avid opacities are also seen in parenchyma of upper lobes of both lungs (D and H—yellow arrow). (*Figure reproduced with permission from:* J Am Coll Cardiol Case Reports. 2024;29(19):102569.)

Her PA angiograms are shown in **Videos 2 and 3**.

Video 2 **Video 3**

The tests for thrombophilia including protein C, protein S, antithrombin 3 deficiency and prothrombin deficiencies, and Factor-5 Leiden were negative.

How should this patient be managed? Compare the CTA with the case 14 to realize the difficulties in the diagnosis. Does she have CTEPH or granulomatous vasculitis or fibrosing mediastinitis or something else?

Pause and think before you click the answer:

Answer: This is a complex case, but then complex cases do occur and we should be able to focus our attention on important aspects. The CT angio picture of CTEPH may be mimicked by Takayasu aortitis, tumors, sarcoid vasculitis, fibrosing mediastinitis, etc. The lymphadenopathy was significant and raised the possibilities of tuberculosis or histoplasmosis. The RA thrombus might be the result of gross RA dilatation. After taking all the investigations into consideration, a decision to operate was taken. At operation, enlarged lymph nodes were found that showed necrotic granuloma on histopathology. She had severe CTEPH in the right PA **(Fig. 16)**.

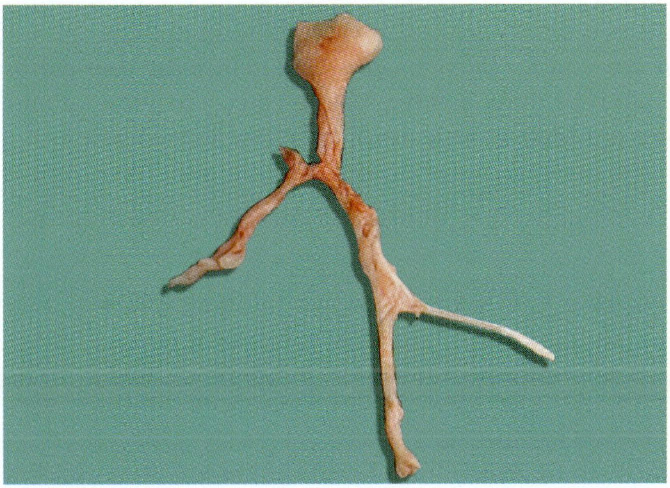

Fig. 16: Intraoperative specimen image showing organized web-like thrombus of the right pulmonary artery suggestive of chronic thromboembolic pulmonary hypertension.

She was given antitubercular therapy and anticoagulation with warfarin and supportive therapy for 6 months, she markedly improved with resolution of PAH.

The dilemma in this case revolve around the diagnosis that can satisfactorily explain the total clinical picture. Finally, she was found to be having two diseases and the relation of tuberculosis with CTEPH in her case remained unknown. Generally, Law of parsimony (explain all things by 1 cause) should be adhered to as a guiding principle, but it may sometimes be overridden after careful clinical considerations. Two diseases could occur in a patient (even though relationship of tuberculosis and CTEPH in this child remains obscure). Tests for thrombophilia were unrevealing.

(*From:* Kadiyani L, Karuru U, Kothari SS, Ramakrishnan S, Gupta SK, Devagouru V, et al. Chronic Thromboembolic Pulmonary Artery Hypertension or Fibrosing Mediastinitis? J Am Coll Cardiol Case Rep. 2024;29(19):102569.)

Learning points: The CTEPH may occur in a young child. Treatable causes of PAH must always be considered.

Sidelights:

1. **What are the risk factors for CTEPH?**
2. **Can CTEPH occur without pulmonary embolism?**
3. **Where in the practice of medicine "the law of parsimony" is often not adhered to?**

(*Sidelights are food for thought—provided to increase your curiosity:* So as a rule, do not read these answers before you try to answer them yourself. The answers provided here are not intended to be exhaustive.)

Answer: Majority of pulmonary emboli resolve with time. CTEPH occurs in <10% of patients with pulmonary embolism. Large emboli, recurrent pulmonary embolism might translate into CTEPH more frequently. However, some factors increase the chances of CTEPH that include patients with splenectomy, hypothyroidism, chronic inflammatory conditions, antiphospholipid antibodies, infected shunts or pacemakers, fibrinogen variants, increased factor 8, or increased Lpa levels. Protein C, protein S deficiency, and other conventional thrombophilic conditions (except those narrated above) are not associated with CTEPH.

- Nearly 25% of patients of CTEPH have no history of deep vein thrombosis (DVT) or pulmonary embolism. In situ thrombosis because of small vessel disease or other causes might represent a different form of CTEPH in some patients and the distinction of in situ thrombi from embolic persistence might be difficult. The pathogenesis of CTEPH is not completely understood.
- Law of parsimony, i.e., explaining the whole process in a particular patient by one cause is a guiding principle for diagnosis in medicine. However, it is often breached in geriatric medicine with the elderly having a multitude of causes and symptoms not necessarily from one disease. This should be recognized, and this important clinical point is also emphasized in geriatric medicine.

CASE

15

Mediastinal Mass in a Cyanosed Boy

"If you do not expect the unexpected you will not find it, for it is not to be reached by search or trail."

—Heraclitus

A 10-year-old boy with posterior mediastinal mass was being considered for surgical resection and was referred because the anesthetic found that the boy was cyanosed. His saturation was 78% on oximeter. The Hemoglobin was 16 g%. The chest X-ray is shown in **Figure 1**.

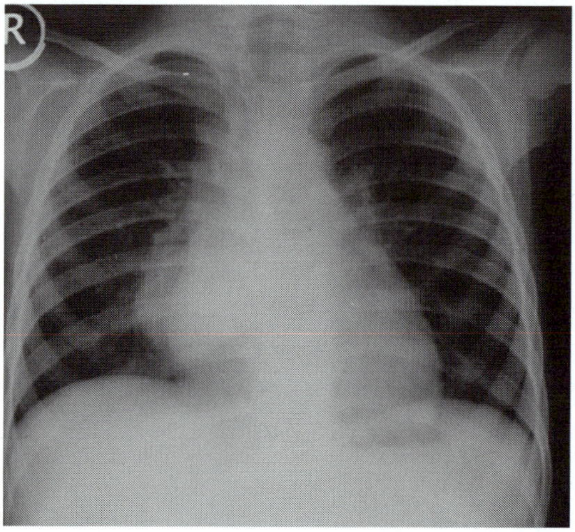

Fig. 1: Chest X-ray.

The echo appeared structurally normal heart. A contrast echo was done that showed microbubbles immediately appearing in the left atrium (LA) after the right ventricular (RV) opacification. The echo is not available, but an angiogram is shown **Video 1**.

Video 1

What is the diagnosis?

Pause and think before you click the answer:

Answers: The patient had a right pulmonary artery (RPA) to left atrial fistula. It is a variant of pulmonary arteriovenous (AV) fistula wherein the RPA drains directly to the LA. This anomaly produces cyanosis, a typical X-ray image, and can be diagnosed by contrast echocardiography. The contract is seen to directly fill LA from the pulmonary artery. In contrast to the typical pulmonary arteriovenous fistula (PAVF), where the contrast appears in the LA after 3–4 beats, the contrast can be seen opacifying LA rather quickly and the communication of RPA to LA is also seen, once the possibility is considered. The fistula might be ligated by surgery without a cardiopulmonary bypass or might be amenable to a device closure.

(*Source:* Ramakrishnan S, Shivdas S, Kothari SS. Trans-septal closure of a right pulmonary artery to left atrial communication. Catheter Cardiovasc Interv. 2010;75(7):1096-9.)

Learning points: The RPA to LA fistula may present with cyanosis, brain abscess, or a mediastinal mass and is easily identified by contrast echo.

Sidelights:

1. **Why systemic AV fistula may produce heart failure, but pulmonary AV fistula does not?**
2. **How do we calculate the amount of shunt through fistula?**

(*Sidelights are food for thought—provided to increase your curiosity:* So as a rule, do not read these answers before you try to answer them yourself. The answers provided here are not intended to be exhaustive.)

Answer: With pulmonary AV fistula, there is no volume overload to the heart. The venous blood that was destined to reach the left ventricular (LV), reaches LV but not saturated. No cardiomegaly is observed. Thus, hypoxia is a problem, whereas with systemic AV fistula, the arterial blood reaches the RV, but the shunted blood is the additional load on the RV and LV. Consequently, there is a biventricular overload and a possibility of heart failure, if the fistula is significant.

- The shunt equation is used to calculate the shunt fraction, i.e., the amount of blood shunted from the cardiac output (Qs/Qt), and typically used in critical care medicine. The equation is very familiar to cardiology residents also as—$Qs/Qt = (CcO_2 - CaO_2)/CcO_2 - CvO_2$ where CcO_2 is pulmonary capillary blood oxygen content, Cao_2 is arterial oxygen content, and CvO_2 is mixed venous oxygen content. However, the difference is that in the case of pulmonary AV fistula, this calculation has to be done while breathing 100% oxygen. Since the fistula might involve only 1 vein, and there may be other heterogeneity in V/Q relationship. 100% oxygen would idealize those discrepancy and represent a concept where the calculated value will represent true shunt. Yes, if there is an additional intracardiac shunt, this equation cannot differentiate the two.

- The video is from a patient with cyanotic heart disease who improved after an operation. However, few years later, his saturation decreased again **(Video 2)**.

Video 2

What is the reason for deterioration?

Answer: The patient had a bilateral bidirectional Glenn operation. Few years later, he developed diffuse PAVF as seen in the angiogram by rapid return of pulmonary artery contrast to pulmonary veins. The reason is the lack of hepatic blood supply to the lungs in a patient of Glenn shunt and the fistulae might disappear if the hepatic venous return is made to circulate through the lungs again!

Now that you have understood PAVF, what if the patient of PAVF has associated pulmonary arterial hypertension (PAH)? Yes, HHT (hereditary hemorrhagic telangiectasia) can have both; but something else is also possible. Read on...

Case 15A: PAH and Pulmonary Arteriovenous Fistula

A 13-year-old boy was having breathlessness for 2 years. On examination, he was in mild congestive heart failure with raised jugular venous pressure (JVP) and a systolic murmur of tricuspid regurgitation (TR). The estimated PA systolic pressure was 60 mm Hg. There were no structural defects. His X-ray is shown below **(Fig. 2)**. His oximetric saturation was 85%. The chest CT showed no significant parenchymal disease, or any PAVF. A contrast echo, however, was suggestive of the PAVF as the contrast appeared in the LA after 3–4 beats. What should be done next in this patient with this clinical profile?

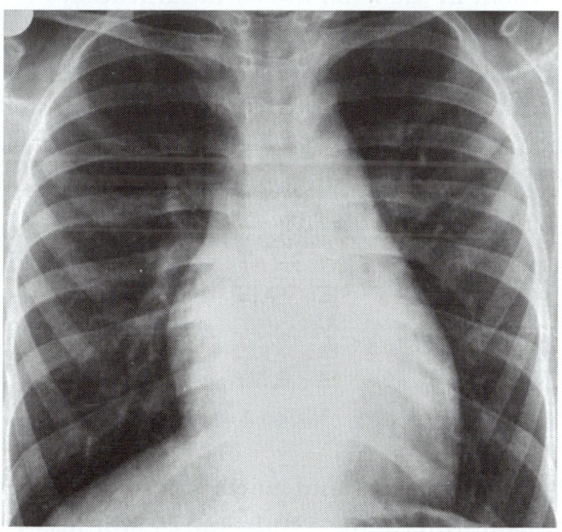

Fig. 2: Chest X-ray.

Pause and think before you click the answer:

Answer: Please see the angiogram before proceeding further. Could you diagnose? **(Video 3)**

Video 3

The combination of PAVF and pulmonary hypertension is highly suspicious of Abernethy syndrome (extrahepatic portosystemic shunt). In this patient, the CT abdomen showed an extracommunication from portal vein to inferior vena cava (IVC). The portosystemic shunt leads to several problems including PAVF, pulmonary hypertension, hepatic angiomas, and hepatic tumors. This communication may be closed by a device or surgically provided there are intrahepatic portal vein radicles. Even if there are few portal radicles present in the liver, the communication between the portal and systemic circulation might be closed and the portal radicles will grow. When there are no intrahepatic portal radicles (type 1 Abernethy syndrome), the communication cannot be closed. Traditionally, in such patients liver transplant may be the only option. However, several reports indicate that the staged closure of the communication might lead to growth of intrahepatic portal radicles as happened in this case also **(Video 4)**.

Video 4

Patients with liver disease and portopulmonary syndrome are well recognized. However, Abernethy syndrome is still less well recognized. Sometimes, the communication may be very unusual and unless strongly suspected, it might be missed. For example, the CT image from a 4-year-old child with a saturation of 85%, and an unexplained episode of incoherent speech of a few hours duration showed a collateral from splenic vein joining to both the internal iliac veins **(Fig. 3)**.

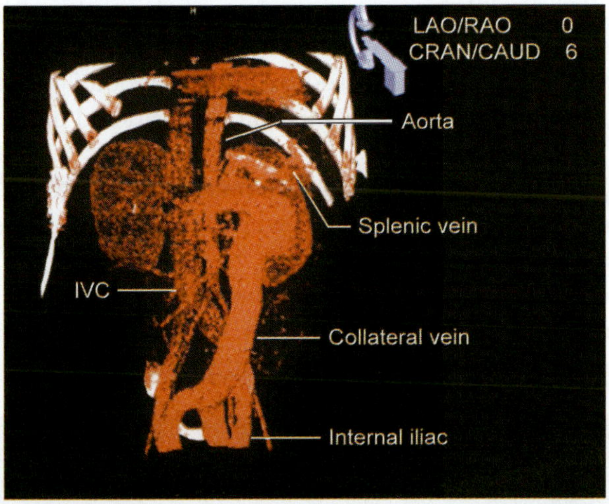

Fig. 3: Reconstructed multiplanar computed tomography image showing the collateral from splenic vein draining into internal iliac veins on both sides after its bifurcation. (Cran: cranial; Caud; caudal; IVC: inferior vena cava)
(*Source:* Senguttuvan NB, Kumar J, Kothari SS. "Treatable" diffuse pulmonary arteriovenous fistula—An unusual cause. Ann Pediatr Cardiol. 2011;4(2):215-6.)

Learning points: In a patient of PAVF or PAH, a raise serum ammonia, episodic encephalopathy, raised serum glutamic-oxaloacetic transaminase/ serum glutamic-pyruvic transaminase (SGOT/SGPT) (uncommon), liver nodules, or liver malignancy should raise suspicion of Abernethy syndrome.

Combination of PAVF and PAH is seen in Abernethy syndrome or liver diseases.

Rarely, an evolution of Abernethy patient from PAVF to disappearance of PAVF and appearance of PAH has been described.

Sidelights:

1. **Abernethy syndrome is associated with which congenital heart disease?**
2. **Should you close PAVF seen in association with PAH?**
3. **Abernethy syndrome and hemangioma—unexplored association.**

(*Sidelights are food for thought—provided to increase your curiosity:* So as a rule, do not read these answers before you try to answer them yourself. The answers provided here are not intended to be exhaustive.)

Answer: In patients with heterotaxy syndrome, Abernethy malformation is seen in up to 10% of patients. Thus, in an unexpected PAH in heterotaxy patient (who often have decreased pulmonary blood flow and pulmonic stenosis), Abernethy syndrome should be considered in an appropriate context.

- PAVF and PAH might be seen in Hereditary hemorrhagic telangiectasia where closure of the fistula might worsen PAH as the closure would increase the afterload.
- Two different patients, both had Abernethy syndrome and typical hemangioma on the external ear! **(Figs. 4A and B)**. (Next time you see such an hemangioma-search for Abernethy syndrome !)

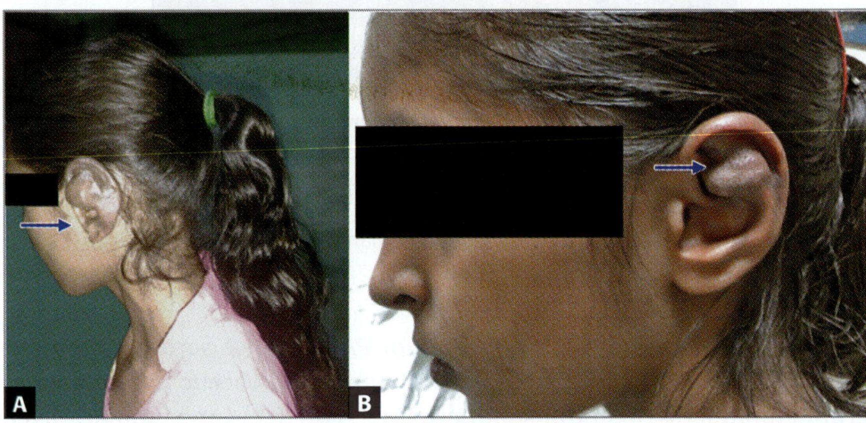

Figs. 4A and B: Ear hemangioma and Abernethy syndrome.
(*Source:* Kothari SS. Hemangioma—A pointer to Abernethy syndrome. Ann Ped Cardiol. 2020:13:269-71.)

CASE

16

Atrial Septal Defect and Ascites

"The three great essentials to achieve anything worthwhile are, first, hard work; second, stick-to-itiveness; and third, common sense."

—Thomas A. Edison

A 14-year-old boy presented with breathlessness and ascites for the last 3 months. He was known to have a hole in the heart since early childhood, but had been generally well. On examination, he had wide fixed second heart sound and congestive heart failure (CHF). His chest X-ray and ECG are shown in **Figures 1 and 2**.

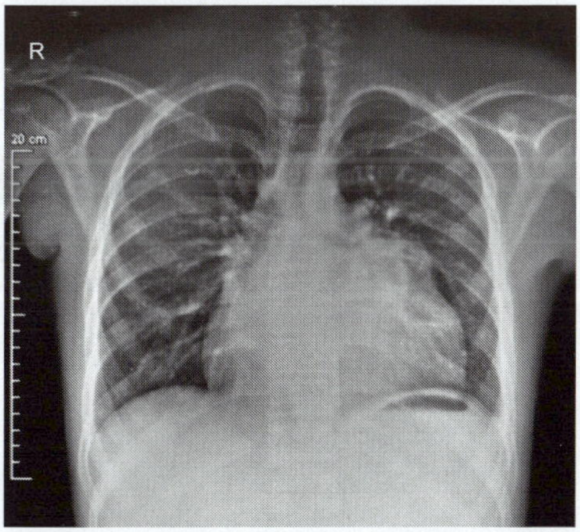

Fig. 1: Chest X-ray showing mild cardiomegaly, pulmonary venous hypertension (PVH) and possible left atrial enlargement.

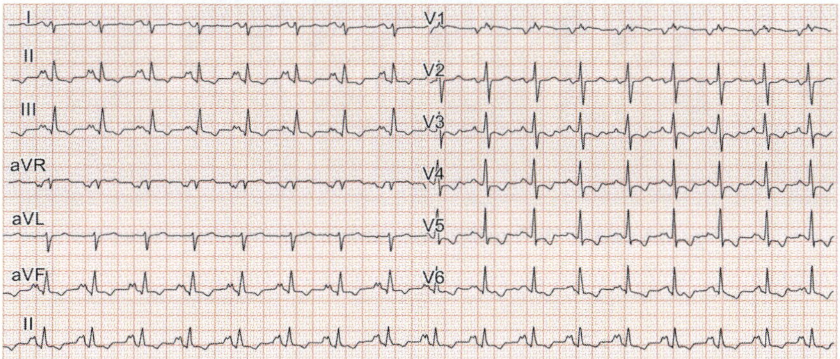

Fig. 2: ECG showing nonspecific ST-T changes, and incomplete RBBB pattern.

The 2D echocardiogram is shown in **Video 1**.

Video 1

The mitral valve (MV) and tricuspid valve (TV) Doppler were as shown in **Figures 3A and B**.

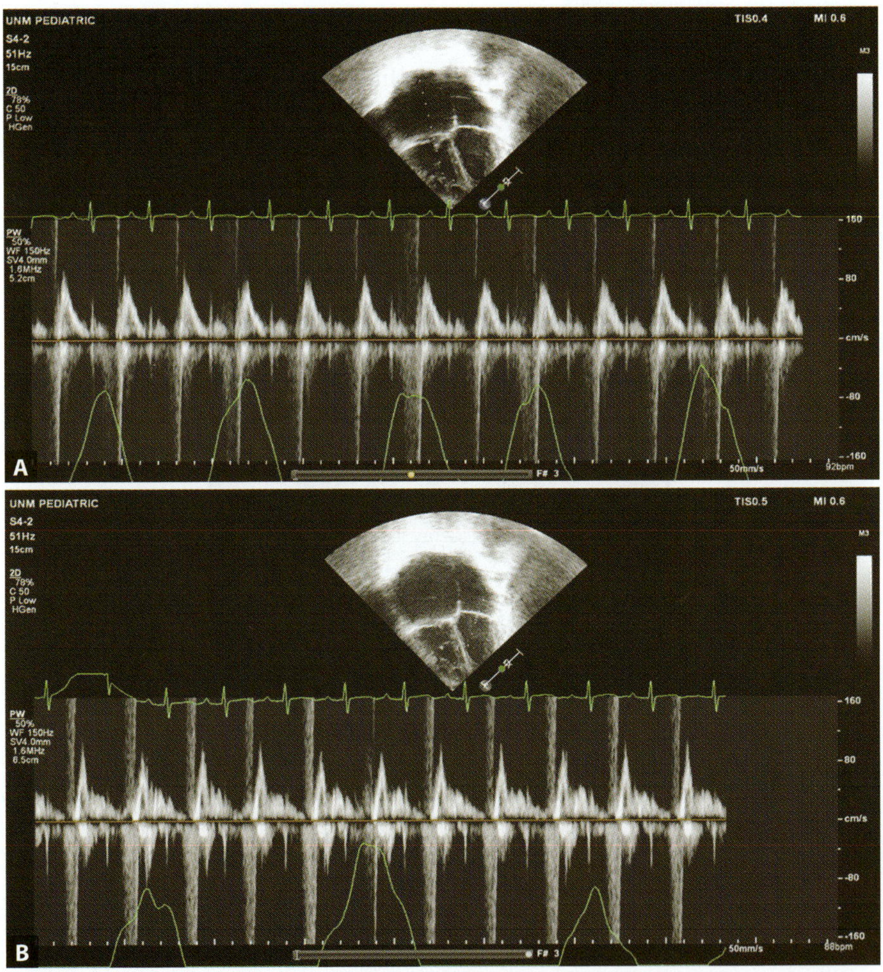

Figs. 3A and B: (A) Doppler across tricuspid; (B) Mitral valves.

A cardiac catheterization was done. The tracings are shown in **Figures 4A and B**).

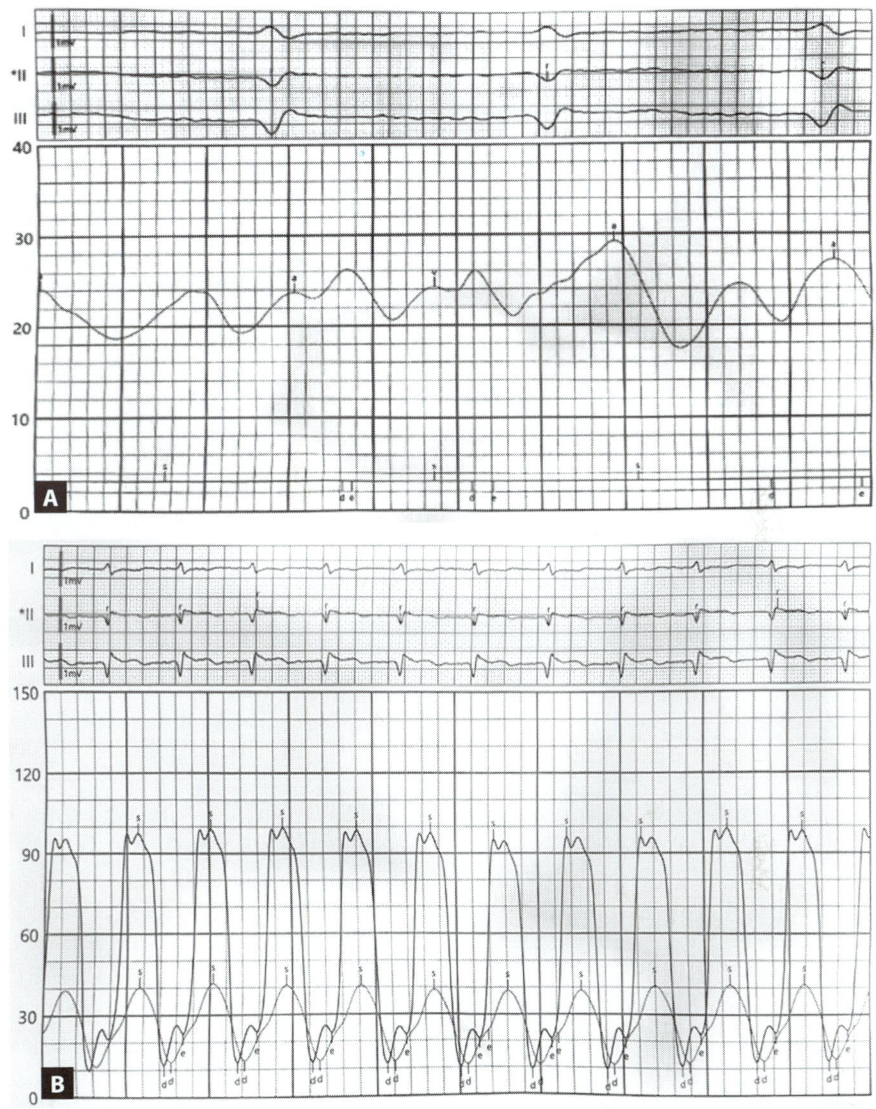

Figs. 4A and B: (A) Right atrial pressure tracings; (B) Simultaneous right and left ventricular pressure tracings.

What is the diagnosis?

Pause and think before you click the answer:

Answer: The patient had an atrial septal defect (ASD) 2° and mitral regurgitation. The echo showed a septal bounce raising the suspicion of chronic constrictive pericarditis (CCP). The right atrial (RA) pressure is markedly elevated. Thus even though there are no respiratory variations in MV/TV Doppler, CCP was suspected. There was no evidence of ventricular interdependence at cardiac cath also, but the end-diastolic pressures were markedly elevated and equalized on right and left side. The cardiac CT also showed thickened pericardium. The patient had a pericardiectomy done, with ASD closure and MV repair and he recovered well. The patient had also received antitubercular therapy for 6 months.

The respiratory variation in MV and TV velocities are very helpful in the diagnosis of CCP. But such variations may be absent in a patient with CCP and ASD, or in patients with markedly increased preload, or arrhythmias.

Markedly increased RA pressures, equalization of ventricular diastolic pressures on cardiac catheterization, and a septal bounce on the echo are the clues for CCP. CT or MRI can be confirmatory, but a normal pericardial thickness may be seen in 15% of patients with CCP. Thus, as always, it is the complete clinical picture, which is diagnostic, and not any one investigation.

Learning points: Respiratory variations in MV or TV Doppler velocity, or evidence of ventricular dependence in cardiac catheterization may be absent in patients with ASD and CCP. Even though, it seems elementary, many such cases have been missed in the real world because of lack of applying common sense.

Sidelights:

1. **What happens with Valsalva maneuver in patients with ASD?**
2. **Is having an ASD advantageous while doing a pulmonary valve balloon dilatation (PVBD) in a patient with severe pulmonic stenosis and tricuspid regurgitation?**
3. **How does having an ASD influence cardiopulmonary bypass?**

(*Sidelights are food for thought—provided to increase your curiosity:* So as a rule, do not read these answers before you try to answer them yourself. The answers provided here are not intended to be exhaustive.)

Answer: Square wave response to Valsalva maneuver is seen in ASD, as the left heart filling does not reduce with the strain. Also seen in patients with CHF, or in CCP, and sometimes in mitral stenosis, and/or aortic stenosis when the increased pulmonary blood volume compensates for the strain induced reduction in preload.

- It is important to remember that while doing a PVBD, if there is an ASD, the left heart preload is maintained when the pulmonary artery is blocked by an inflated balloon and therefore no hypotension may occur, but the right-to-left shunt can cause severe desaturation. Thus central nervous system (CNS) injury might result from prolonged inflation of balloon across pulmonary valve from hypoxemia, while there would be no hypotension. Such cases have been reported.
- This is to bring to the attention the problems of air embolism during bypass. The ASD provide an easy route for systemic air embolism in many situations in cardiac surgery whenever a possibility exists for the event to occur. Hence, presence or absence of ASD must be clear before any cardiopulmonary bypass surgery (one example is that the anesthetist maintains a positive pressure during placement of atrial/caval cannula, the preload is kept sufficient so that RA pressure is not subatmospheric, otherwise air can get into systemic circuit).

CASE

17

Postoperative Congestive Heart Failure in a Child

"The simple things are also the most extraordinary things, and only the wise can see them."

—Paulo Coelho

A 3-year-old child had complex cyanotic congenital heart disease (CHD) with unbalanced atrioventricular septal defect (AVSD) and double outlet right ventricle (DORV) with pulmonary arterial hypertension (PAH). There was left AV valve stenosis, a small primum atrial septal defect (ASD), and a patent ductus arteriosus (PDA). After cardiac catheterization, she underwent an atrial septectomy, PDA ligation, and a pulmonary artery (PA) band. The child improved significantly symptomatically. However, she again presented 2 years later with progressive ascites and severe congestive heart failure. Her chest X-ray at this presentation is shown in **Figure 1**. The echo videos are shown in **Videos 1 to 3**. There was no significant change in the valve regurgitation or ventricular contractility. The PA band gradient of 50 mm Hg was unchanged. No other intercurrent illness was reported. A CT scan reported no significant abnormality other than the congenital defects **(Fig. 2)**. What could be the diagnosis? A cardiac catheterization showed a right atrial mean of 20 mm Hg and ventricular end diastolic pressure of 20 mm Hg.

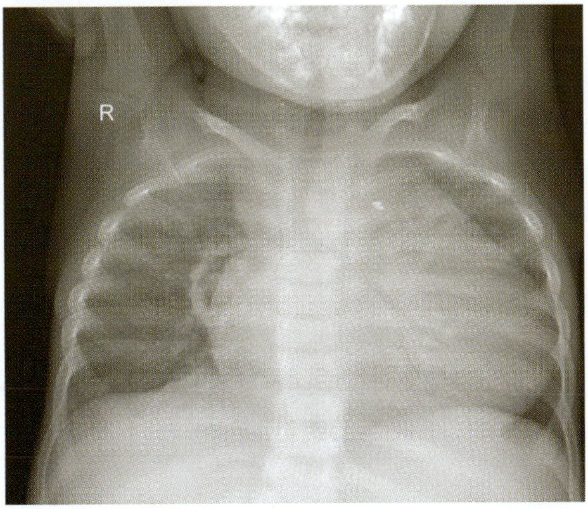

Fig. 1: Chest X-ray of the patient with heart failure.

Video 1 **Video 2** **Video 3**

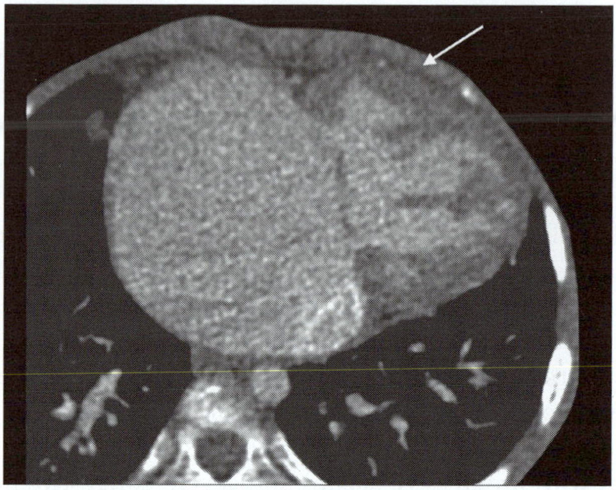

Fig. 2: Computed tomography (CT) scan showing normal thickness of pericardium (arrow).

What is the diagnosis? Likely possibilities?

Pause and think before you click the answer:

Answer: In the absence of any other abnormality like worsening of the valvar regurgitation or decrease in ventricular contractility, constrictive pericarditis was suspected despite a normal CT report and cardiomegaly. At operation, adherent and thickened pericardium was found. Histology showed dense fibrosis, focal thickening, and chronic inflammatory infiltrate. The child improved markedly over the next few weeks and later underwent a bidirectional Glenn operation as well.

This case illustrates that discrimination is needed in interpreting the investigation reports. Although chronic constrictive pericarditis (CCP) with normal thickness of pericardium occurs in 15% of CCP cases, it seemed unlikely following a PA band and septectomy surgery. The chest X-ray seems most unlike a CCP X-ray. However, the clinical course left no other option for the diagnosis; and the postoperative course and the histology **(Figs. 3A and B)** vindicated a very unusual diagnosis.

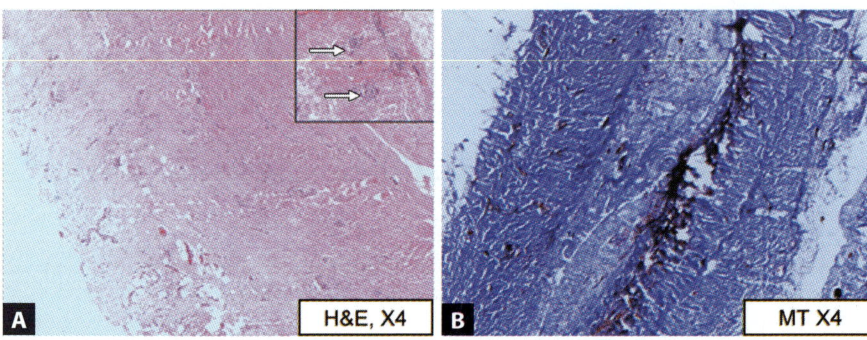

Figs. 3A and B: Histopathology of the excised pericardium. Pericardium showing: (A) Dense fibrosis and hyalinization with focal chronic inflammatory cell infiltration (inset, arrows); (B) Masson trichrome stain shows fibrosis (blue).

(*Source:* Deepti S, Gupta SK, Ramakrishnan S, Talwar S, Kothari SS. Constrictive pericarditis following open-heart surgery in a child. Ann Pediatr Cardiol. 2016;9(1):68-71.)

Learning points: Postoperative CCP may occur after a closed heart surgery. Discrimination is needed to separate wheat from chaff when all investigations are unrevealing or contradictory.

Sidelights: What is the mechanism of ascites praecox, i.e., ascites earlier than edema seen in CCP?

(*Sidelights are food for thought—provided to increase your curiosity:* So as a rule, do not read these answers before you try to answer them yourself. The answers provided here are not intended to be exhaustive.)

Answer: Ascites praecox, i.e., ascites earlier than edema typically occurs in chronic constrictive pericarditis, and with severe tricuspid valve disease with markedly increased right atrial (RA) pressures. Curiously, in many of these patients, the pedal edema is disproportionately little. The fact that ascites occur earlier than edema is explained by many as the hepatic veins are also constricted at their entry and resultant hepatic congestion leads to lymph exudation into peritoneum. Accompanying hypoalbuminemia, sometimes tricuspid regurgitation directly into the hepatic veins, and associated peritoneal inflammation are other hypotheses. However, the mechanism of disproportionate ascites has not been adequately understood.

CASE

18

Recurrent Pericardial Effusion

"To rise from error to truth is rare and beautiful".

—Victor Hugo

A 4-year-old girl was referred because of recurrent hemorrhagic pericardial effusion. The child had an insidious onset of breathlessness for 6 months and had episodes of lower respiratory tract infection. Pericardial effusion was detected on chest X-ray and hemorrhagic fluid was aspirated. She was started on antitubercular drugs with steroids, but her condition did not improve significantly. The patient had normal development in her early infancy and normal growth prior to this illness. There was no family history of heart disease, developmental defects, tuberculosis, or connective tissue disorder. On examination, she was in mild respiratory distress. Her chest X-ray is shown in **Figure 1**.

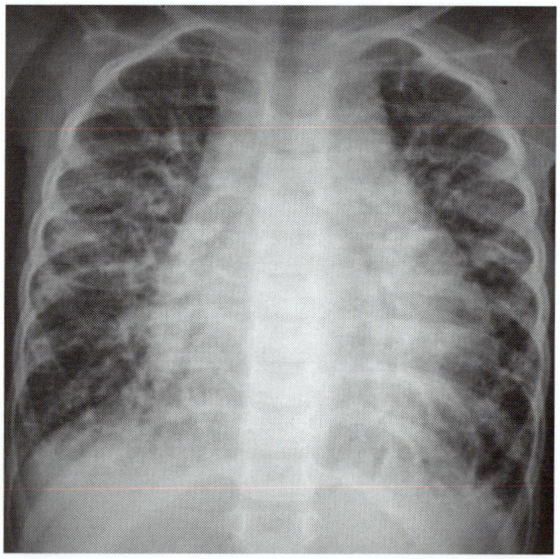

Fig. 1: Chest X-ray showing streaky lung fields in addition to smooth mild cardiomegaly.

Her hemoglobin was 8.7 g/dL, and her total leukocyte count (TLC) was 10,600/mm^3 with 65% neutrophils. An echocardiogram showed a large pericardial effusion (2.0 cm circumferentially) with evidence of tamponade. A total of 300 mL of hemorrhagic pericardial fluid was aspirated with a pigtail catheter in the pericardium. The pericardial fluid showed numerous red blood cells (RBCs), but no malignant cells were found. The adenosine deaminase in the fluid was not elevated. The bacterial and fungal cultures were sterile. Results of her abdominal ultrasound examination were normal. The fluid in the pericardium reaccumulated within weeks of drainage. The antitubercular treatment and steroids were stopped. Meanwhile, results of her thyroid function tests were normal. Her rheumatoid factor, antinuclear antibodies, and antineutrophilic cytoplasmic antibodies were negative. Tests for human immunodeficiency virus (HIV), hepatitis B surface antigen (HBsAg), and hepatitis C were negative and immunoglobulins were normal. A high-resolution computed tomography (HRCT) scan showed peculiar diffuse polygonal lobular architect **(Fig. 2)** and soft tissue mediastinal mass.

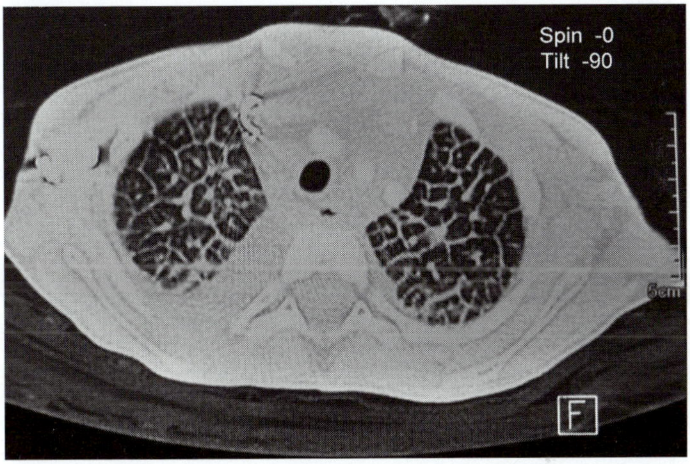

Fig. 2: High-resolution computed tomography image of the chest shows thickened interlobular septae with typical polygonal architecture.

A needle biopsy of the mediastinal mass revealed only fat and connective tissues. Repeated pericardial fluid analyses for malignant cells were negative. Her platelet counts were 50–70,000/mm^3 on multiple occasions. She also tested negative for disseminated intravascular coagulation (DIC). Her bone marrow was normal.

What is the diagnosis?

Pause and think before you click the answer:

Answer: A skeletal survey showed lytic lesions in the long bones that clinched the diagnosis **(Fig. 3)**.

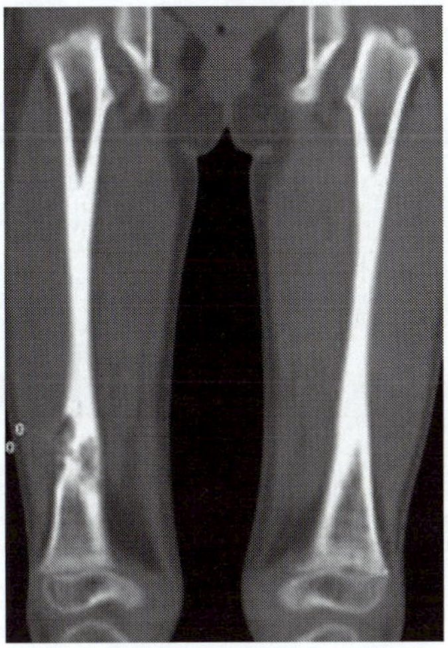

Fig. 3: A coronal computed tomography shows an osteolytic lesion in the lower third of the right femur.

This rare case is presented to highlight the approach to recurrent pericardial effusion. The approach to recurrent hemorrhagic pericardial effusion may be difficult. Tuberculosis, viral pericarditis, neoplasm, connective tissue disorders, and drugs are typically responsible in the majority of cases. Recurrent chylothorax is better known in children and has multiple causes. The effusion in this child was hemorrhagic and was recurrent. The presence of a soft tissue mass, a typical CT picture, and the lytic lesions in the bone led to the diagnosis of Gorham's disease. The child had a hemangiolymphangiomatosis (Gorham's disease) involving multiple systems. Diffuse lymphangiomatosis is a rare, nonmalignant but locally infiltrative multisystem disease that may involve any tissue except the brain. The thorax, bones, and spleen are typically involved. The clinical course is highly variable, but disease occurrence and lung involvement in children suggest a poorer prognosis. Due to recurrent pericardial effusion, an open pericardiectomy was done and the lung biopsy at that time showed the lymphangiohemangiomatosis **(Fig. 4)**. Unfortunately, the child succumbed after a few months of illness.

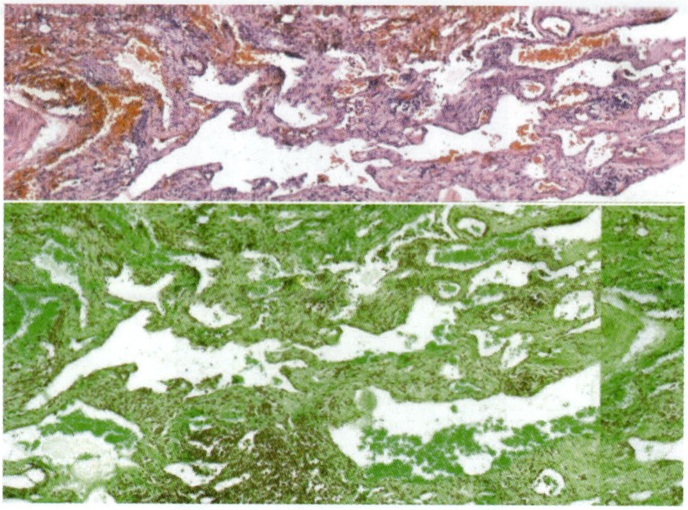

Fig. 4: Lung biopsy (hematoxylin and eosin imaging) shows multiple proliferating vascular spaces lined with endothelium infiltrating the interstitium. Lymphoid tissue is seen in the stroma. Some of the spaces contain blood. (The lining cells were CD 31+ which is a marker for endothelial cells but does not distinguish lymphatic from vascular endothelium.)

(*Source:* Kothari SS, Sharma S, Bhatt K, Ray R, Bakhshi S, Chowdhury U. Recurrent hemorrhagic pericardial effusion in a child due to diffuse lymphangiohemangiomatosis: a case report. J Med Case Rep. 2010;4:62.)

Learning points: Although uncommon manifestations of common diseases are more common than uncommon diseases, rare disorders do occur. Gorham's disease is a less well-understood multisystem disease that may present with soft tissue masses and lytic bone lesions. When faced with a clinically difficult situation, it is well to keep looking in all directions, and updating and revisiting the investigations as this case teaches us.

Sidelights:

1. **What are the causes of milky pleural effusions?**
2. **What are the causes of lymphedema?**

(*Sidelights are food for thought—provided to increase your curiosity:* So as a rule, do not read these answers before you try to answer them yourself. The answers provided here are not intended to be exhaustive.)

Answer: Milky pleural effusion might result from empyema, chylothorax, or cholesterol effusion (pseudochylous or chyliform effusions). It is important to have a clear understanding of these disorders so that an appropriate management strategy may be employed when faced with the situation. On centrifugation, empyema will separate out into clear and cloudy fluids whereas both chylothorax and pseudochylothorax will remain milky. Typically, the clinical contexts are different. Chylothorax is important to cardiologists as it may be seen in their patients after cardiac surgery, or uncommonly in patients with heart failure, cirrhosis, nephrotic syndrome, etc. Chylothorax is identified by triglycerides >110 mg/dL, lymphocytes >50%, and a protein concentration that is variable, but commonly lactate dehydrogenase (LDH) levels are in the transudative range. Occasionally, chylous fluid may coexist with other etiology of pleural effusion and may have a complicated fluid picture, but the presence of chylomicrons in the fluid is diagnostic of chylothorax. It is good to remember that milky appearance is seen only in half of the patients with chylothorax, so pleural fluid should be investigated with triglycerides in clinically appropriate situations for chylothorax even if the fluid is not milky. Pseudochylous effusion will always have higher cholesterol than triglycerides in the fluid, and triglycerides are usually <110 mg/dL. Such effusions are seen in chronic empyema, tuberculosis, or rheumatoid arthritis and are associated with thickened pleura and lung entrapment. Fluids have a satin-like appearance and have cholesterol crystals. The pathogenesis of cholesterol effusion is unclear, but therapy often needs decortication. Thus, management pathways are quite different.

- Apart from filariasis, lymphedema might occur in myxedema, lymph node obstructions in tumors, postsurgery compromising lymph flow, congenital lymphatic abnormalities with Noonan syndrome, Turner syndrome, yellow nail syndrome, and Milroy disease. **Figure 5** shows a case of Turner syndrome with lymphedema that was unnecessarily investigated for many diseases because of not recognizing the association.

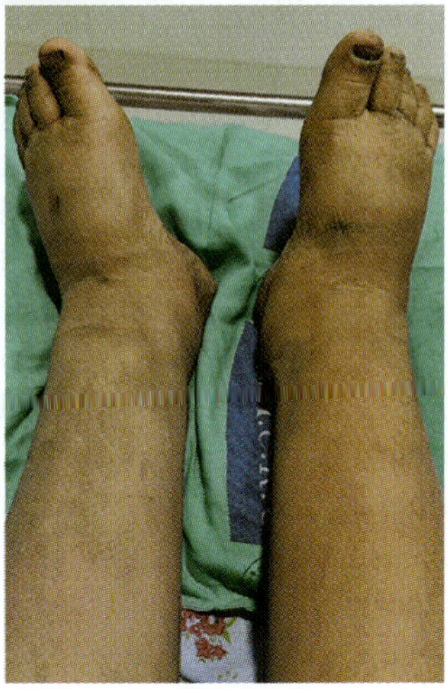

Fig. 5: Lymphedema in a 10-year-old boy with Noonan syndrome.

CASE

19

Pericardial Effusion in an Elderly Lady

"The mind is not a vessel to be filled, but a fire to be kindled".

—Plutarch

A 70-year-old lady had an old anterior wall myocardial infarction 5 years earlier. She was receiving treatment for hypertension, and hypothyroidism and was generally well. She now had complaints of increasing breathlessness for the last 2 months and lower abdominal dull ache. Her breathlessness worsened, and she was found to have pericardial effusion. The fluid was drained and she was started on antitubercular therapy empirically, but she continued to be symptomatic despite the therapy. Repeat evaluation showed large pleural and pericardial effusion. Her ECG and chest X-ray are shown in **Figures 1 and 2**.

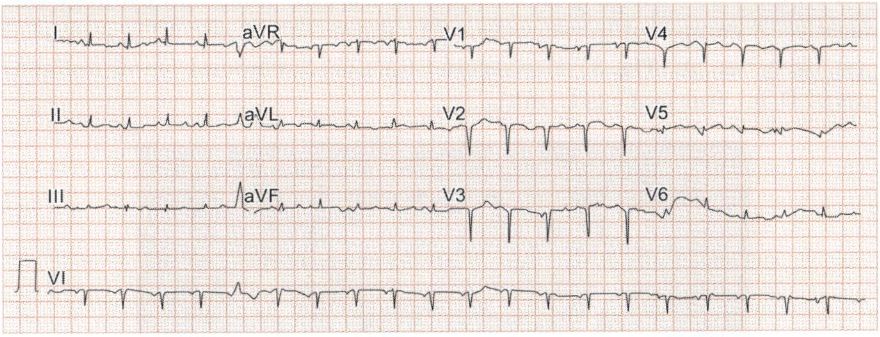

Fig. 1: ECG showing low voltages and poor progression of R wave.

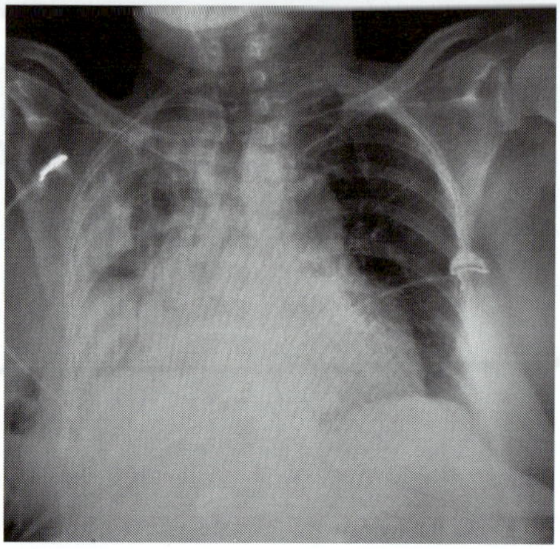

Fig. 2: Chest X-ray showing pleural and pericardial effusion.

Her echo showed pericardial effusion, apical hypokinesia, and multiple left ventricular (LV) thrombi.

An intercostal tube drainage was placed for the pleural fluid and pericardiocentesis was also done. The pericardial fluid was exudative, and adenosine deaminase was normal. There were 260 cells/mm^3 with 60% lymphocytes. GeneXpert for tuberculosis and malignant cytology was negative. A computed tomography (CT) abdomen showed a large ovarian cyst, likely benign **(Fig. 3)**. Her serum CEA 125 (carcinoembryonic antigen) was 97 U/mL (normal <35 U/mL).

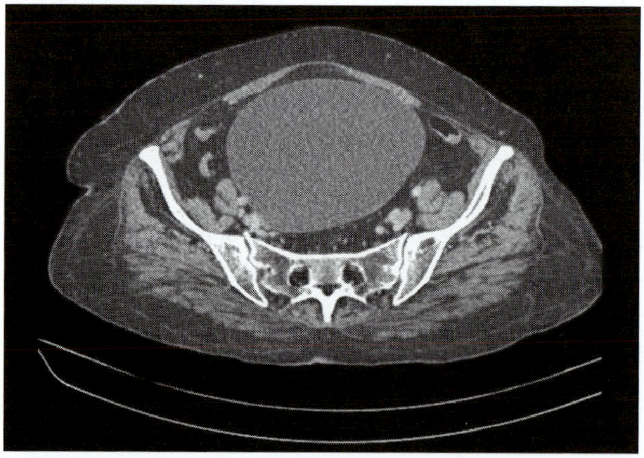

Fig. 3: Computed tomography (CT) of abdomen and pelvis showing 101 × 106 × 126 mm sized well-defined rounded minimally peripherally enhancing cystic lesion in right ovary likely benign cystic ovarian lesion.

Recurrent pericardial effusion despite antitubercular therapy and negative cytology for malignant cells made the diagnosis difficult.

What is the diagnosis?

Pause and think before you click the answer:

Answer: Meigs syndrome is a well-known cause of pleural effusion with a benign ovarian fibroma. (Pleural effusion with other ovarian cysts and masses is often termed as pseudo-Meigs syndrome; the two are used interchangeably here). A pericardial effusion due to Meigs syndrome is rarely recognized. The effusion in Meigs syndrome might be transudative or exudative. We diagnosed Meigs syndrome as a cause of her pericardial effusion after all investigations, and she underwent ovarian cyst removal. Unfortunately, she had a brainstem stroke from the LV thrombi despite anticoagulation and she died. The autopsy was not done; therefore, the assertion remains somewhat unproven, but the case is presented here for stimulating the thought that we need to go out of the heart sometimes to diagnose a cardiac condition!

Learning points: Meigs syndrome may present with transudative, or mostly an exudative pericardial effusion. The mechanism of pericardial or pleural effusion in Meigs syndrome is not known but exudation of fluids from the mass, lymphatic obstruction by the tumor causing a leak of fluid, and more recently, inflammatory cytokines such as VEGF, IL-6, and fibroblast growth factor that increase capillary permeability have been incriminated. It is imperative to exclude malignancy first, and the diagnosis is established by the disappearance of the effusion after the removal of the mass.

Sidelights:

1. **Catamenial pneumothorax is known. Catamenial pericardial effusion is not yet reported. Do you think it might occur?**
2. **Pseudo-pseudo Meigs syndrome is also worth keeping in mind as a cause of pericardial effusion.**
3. **What are the fluid characteristics of pericardial effusion in hypothyroidism?**

(*Sidelights are food for thought—provided to increase your curiosity:* So as a rule, do not read these answers before you try to answer them yourself. The answers provided here are not intended to be exhaustive.)

Answer: You have to answer. Hint: Pericardial endometriosis is reported.

- Pseudo-pseudo Meigs is a more recently recognized manifestation of systemic lupus erythematosus (SLE) with pleural effusion, ascites, and raised CA-125 that may present even before other manifestations of SLE. Pericardial effusion is not yet reported, but it may just be a matter of time, like this case.
- Hypothyroidism may cause large pericardial effusion and only rarely cardiac tamponade due to slowly developing fluid. The pathogenesis is attributed to a change in capillary permeability to albumin and slow lymphatic drainage. Thus, generally, pericardial effusion with hypothyroidism shows high protein content like an exudate with few cells only. Most often, even large pericardial effusion resolves with the treatment of hypothyroidism, and hence the fluid should not be drained.

If this did not appear very interesting, see the bonus case.

Case 19A: Cardiogenic Shock in a 5-Year-Old Child

A 5-year-old child had progressive breathlessness for 1 year and had rapid deterioration in the last 5 days. She presented to casualty with severe respiratory distress and a thready pulse. Her heart rate was 144 beats/min, and the systolic blood pressure was only 50 mm Hg. She appeared in gross congestive heart failure with jugular venous pressure (JVP) markedly elevated. Information from her echo is shown in **Figures 4A and B** and in **Videos 1 and 2**.

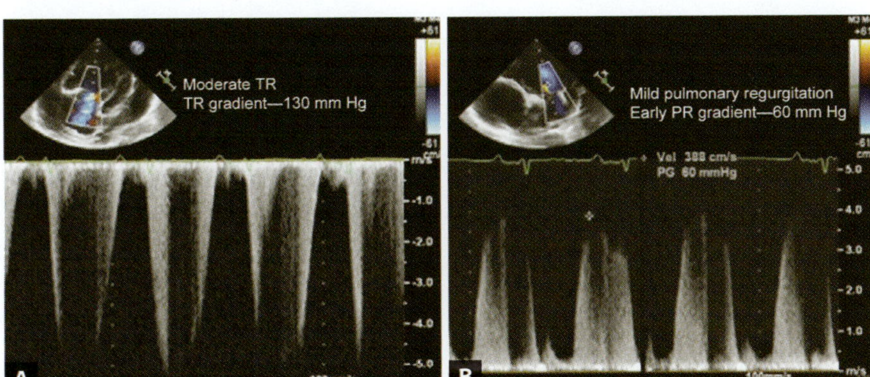

Figs. 4A and B: The echocardiograms.

Video 1 Video 2

What is the diagnosis?

Pause and think before you click the answer:

Answer: The echo shows cardiac tamponade with only left heart collapse. Pulsus paradoxus was not apparent as the pulse was thready and blood pressure was only 50 mm Hg. The patient had severe pulmonary artery hypertension (PAH) and was in gross right heart failure. There was severe tricuspid regurgitation with suprasystemic pulmonary artery pressures. No right atrial or right ventricular collapse is seen because of right ventricular hypertrophy. However, the left ventricle and left atrial collapse are seen. Regional tamponade is more typically seen in postoperative patients. Tamponade in patients with severe PAH is a sinister finding. The pericardiocentesis is often not rewarding and should be avoided as far as possible. In this patient, after tapping, there was an immediate rise in systolic pressure and relief from dyspnea. However, she died after 8 hours due to low cardiac output and right heart failure.

(*Source:* Varghese MJ, Kothari SS. Cardiac tamponade with only left heart collapse in a child with severe pulmonary artery hypertension. Echocardiography. 2013;30(8):E263-4.)

Learning points: Cardiac tamponade may occur without RA/RV collapse.

Sidelights:

1. **Can a patient with cardiac tamponade have hypertension?**
2. **What is pericardial decompression syndrome?**
3. **Which cardiac tamponade should not have pericardiocentesis?**
4. **Does a low-pressure tamponade patient show RA/RV collapse?**

(*Sidelights are food for thought—provided to increase your curiosity:* So as a rule, do not read these answers before you try to answer them yourself. The answers provided here are not intended to be exhaustive.)

Answer: It is erroneous to think that a heart in tamponade cannot generate enough pressure to have hypertension. Thus, the diagnosis of tamponade must not be discounted based on arterial pressure readings only. In some series of cardiac tamponade patients presenting to emergency services, up to 30% had systemic hypertension!

- Sudden removal of large amounts of fluid from the pericardium, paradoxically leads to hypotension and shock/pulmonary edema after initial improvement in patients of cardiac tamponade, usually in large chronic effusion. It is rather uncommon and should not make anyone reluctant to drain the pericardium during tamponade. However, large volumes should not be drained (not >800 mL or so possibly) rapidly. The pathophysiology of this syndrome is not well understood and might relate to sudden changes in preload/afterload matching and ventricular interdependence during the transition.
- Pericardiocentesis might worsen the patients of aortic dissection with tamponade; hence, it must be carefully considered in this setting, in dire emergency, only a small amount of drainage might tide over the crisis.
- Low-pressure tamponade patient is in tamponade, only his overall status of dehydration, or low intravascular volumes and low intrapericardial pressures make the recognition difficult. However, they would have RA and RV collapse that could become more prominent after intravenous fluid replacement.

CASE

20

Dilated Cardiomyopathy in a Child

"It's not what you look at that matters, it's what you see."

—Henry David Thoreau

A 9-year-old child was referred with the diagnosis of dilated cardiomyopathy (DCM) for further management. Clinical examination showed a pulse of 92 beats/min, blood pressure 130/100 mm Hg, cardiomegaly, and raised jugular venous pressure (JVP). On auscultation, there was LVS3, but no murmur. Peripheral pulses were equal. Echo showed a dilated left ventricle with an ejection fraction (EF) of 30%. Mild ventricular hypertrophy was there. A history of phlyctenular keratoconjunctivitis and skin rash was there 2 months prior to the onset of the illness. Her ESR was 45 mm/h. The chest X-ray is shown in **Figure 1**.

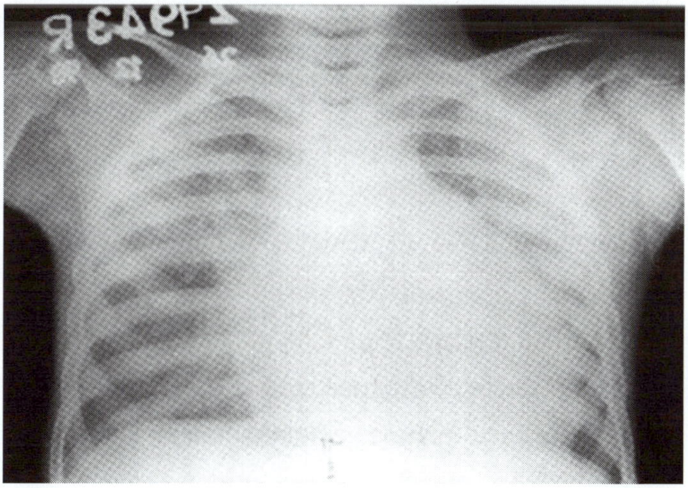

Fig. 1: Chest X-ray showing cardiomegaly and pulmonary venous hypertension (PVH).

What should be done further other than the treatment of heart failure?

Pause and think before you click the answer:

Answer: She underwent an aortogram that showed bilateral renal artery stenosis (**Figs. 2A and B**). She was treated with steroids, antitubercular drugs, and subsequently renal angioplasty. Her left ventricular (LV) function recovered over a few months. Takayasu aortoarteritis often masquerades as DCM. A careful history, asymmetric peripheral pulses, an abdominal bruit, and hypertension would point to the correct diagnosis in the majority of the cases. Weak left subclavian (most common artery involved), or weak femorals (mimicking coarctation of aorta) are found on physical examination. Occasionally as seen in this case, symmetric pulses are there. Sometimes, hypertension might be missed because of the vascular narrowing on that side or might get obtunded with the onset of ventricular dysfunction. Therefore, a high index of suspicion in the appropriate context is needed to identify this

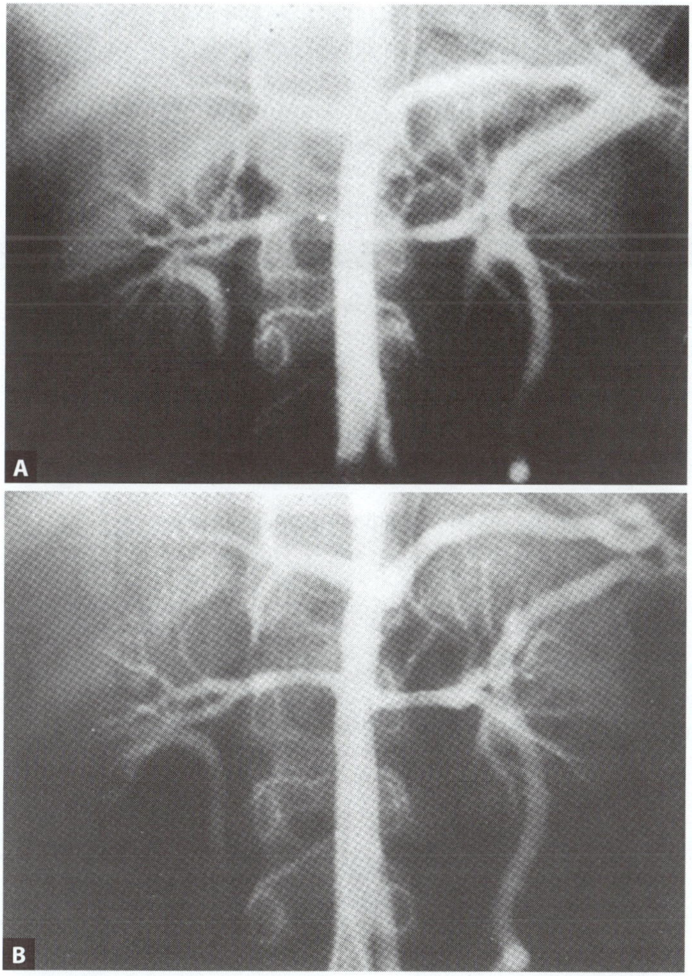

Figs. 2A and B: Aortogram before and after renal artery dilatation.

treatable cause of ventricular dysfunction. In this child, peripheral pulses were symmetrical, but hypertension, mild left ventricular hypertrophy (LVH), and a history of Phlyctenular conjunctivitis were suspicious of Takayasu aortitis. Sick-looking child with increased ESR further raised the clinical suspicion. Familiarity with the disease and the clinical context is important since we do not always do an aortogram for the diagnosis of hypertension in children! Takayasu aortoarteritis might also cause valvular regurgitation, myocarditis, coronary artery involvement, and pulmonary artery involvement.

- This 4-year-old boy with similar renal artery stenosis **(Fig. 3)** was not treated with steroids as his examination showed something else that took the diagnosis away from aortoarteritis. Any guess?

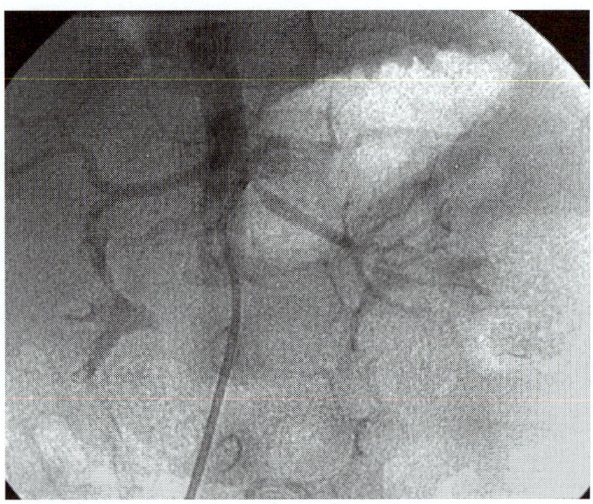

Fig. 3: Another patient with renal artery stenosis.

Pause and think before you click the answer:

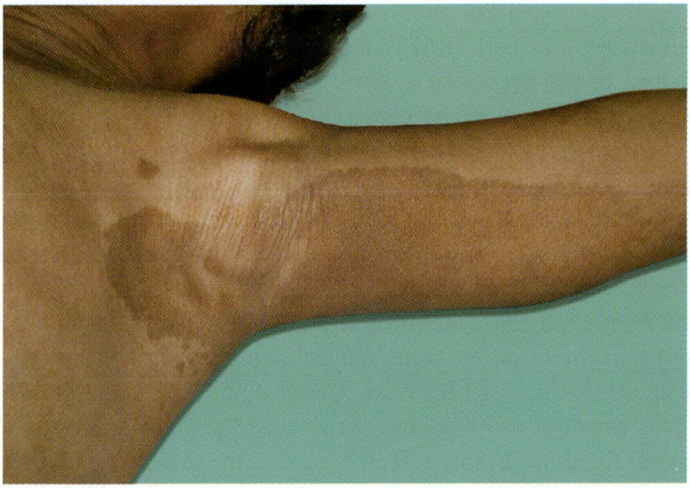

Fig. 4: Large Café-au-lait spots in a patient with neurofibromatosis and renal artery stenosis.

This patient had neurofibromatous involvement of renal arteries causing renal artery stenosis. The angiographic picture can be very similar to Takayasu arteritis. She had multiple large café-au-lait spots as a pointer to the diagnosis of neurofibromatous RAS **(Fig. 4)**. Her cardiac function was normal.

(*Source:* Malav IC, Kothari SS. Renal artery stenosis due to neurofibromatosis. Ann Pediatr Cardiol. 2009;2(2):167-9.)

These two cases illustrate the importance of raising the appropriate clinical context and the importance of making a correct clinical diagnosis.

Learning points: Takayasu aortoarteritis is an important cause of ventricular dysfunction in some parts of the world. The angiographic picture of Takyasu aortitis might be very similar to that of neurofibromatous involvement of the aorta/renal arteries. Ventricular function might recover as the hypertension is better controlled with the treatment of renal artery stenosis.

Sidelights: Why angiotensin-converting enzyme (ACE) inhibitors are the drug of choice for the treatment of unilateral renal artery stenosis (RAS) but contraindicated in bilateral RAS?

(*Sidelights are food for thought—provided to increase your curiosity:* So as a rule, do not read these answers before you try to answer them yourself. The answers provided here are not intended to be exhaustive.)

Answer: ACEi are excellent antihypertensive agents, especially in patients with renal artery stenosis (RAS) since they have high renin-angiotensin hypertension. In the presence of RAS, the glomerular filtration rate (GFR) might fall with the use of ACEi as they abolish angiotensin-mediated efferent vasoconstriction. This effect may be dependent on the levels of angiotensin in the body and when there is bilateral RAS, a decline in GFR might precipitate renal failure. Such an event is not seen in unilateral RAS as the GFR is maintained in the other kidney, but the ipsilateral kidney might suffer. If the RAS is very severe (say >95% for example), the GFR fall might be significant. As such, there is no fundamental difference between 1- or 2-sided RAS except that the manifest renal failure is not seen in unilateral RAS. The fate of ipsilateral kidneys with severe RAS and ACEi use has not been widely studied. It is prudent to be aware of this and use ACEi cautiously in RAS. Nevertheless, ACEi are highly effective agents in RAS and must be utilized. Most patients with bilateral RAS are also able to tolerate and benefit from the use of ACEi, unless the RAS is severe.

Unusual occurrence of renal artery thrombosis after ACEi in unilateral RAS; probably triggered by the very tight narrowing and significant fall of blood pressure with ACEi (**Figs. 5A and B**).

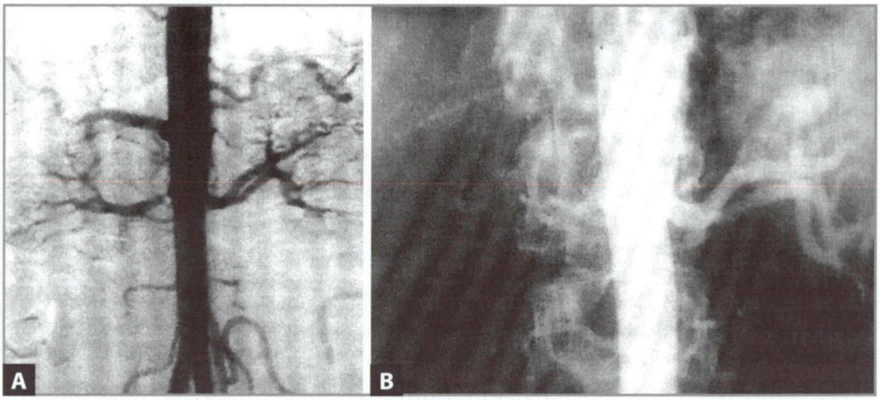

Figs. 5A and B: (A) DSA shows tight RAS. The patient planned for balloon dilatation. Blood pressure controlled with ACEi; (B) Angiogram after 1 week shows occlusion of renal artery!

(*Source:* Kothari SS, Sharma S, Sharma M, Saxena A. Enalapril-induced renal artery thrombosis in unilateral renal artery stenosis. Indian Heart J. 1997;49(2):192-4.)

CASE

21

Heart Failure and Mitral Regurgitation in an Elderly Lady

"He who is seeking knowledge should give up comfort,
He who is seeking comfort should give up learning knowledge,
As the knowledge seeker cannot get comfort and a comfort seeker cannot learn knowledge."

—Chanakya

An 82-year-old previously healthy lady presented with acute onset breathlessness of 3 days duration. She was known hypertensive for 10 years. There was no chest pain or ST segment changes in ECG, and trop I was not elevated. The chest X-ray is shown in **Figure 1**. Her pulse was 100 beats/min, BP was 220/100 mm Hg, oximeter showed 91% saturation, and a pan systolic murmur of mitral regurgitation (MR) was heard. There was no fever. Routine investigations including renal function test (RFT), liver function test (LFT), and thyroid functions were normal. A CART done through the right radial artery showed insignificant coronary artery disease. NT-pro BNP was 2,695 pg/mL.

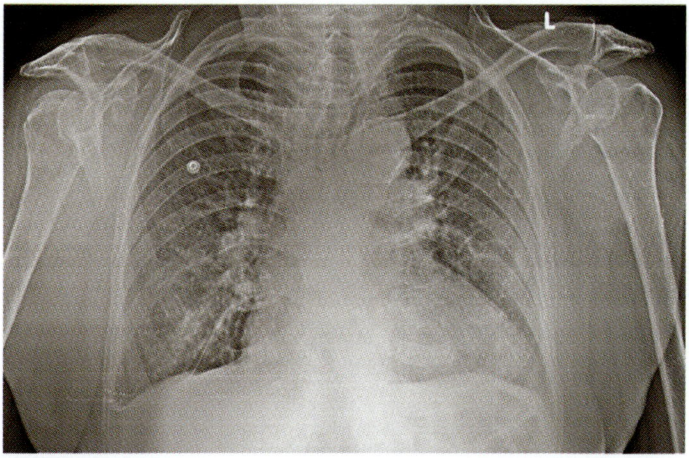

Fig. 1: Chest X-ray showing cardiomegaly and unfolding of aorta.

Echocardiogram showed severe MR **(Video 1)**. Normal left ventricular (LV) systolic functions and estimated pulmonary artery (PA) systolic pressure of 80 mm Hg.

Video 1

After usual therapy for heart failure with diuretics, angiotensin receptor blockers (ARB), and β-blockers, she was being considered for a mitraclip for the severe MR. But her MR almost disappeared. (Why?)**(Video 2)**

Video 2

She had malena from duodenal ulcer requiring blood transfusion and hemoclip. She recovered from malena, but she developed oliguria, worsening of renal functions, and breathlessness. Abdominal ultrasound showed normal renal artery flow and bilateral normal-sized kidneys with maintained corticomedullary differentiation. Repeated urine analyses were normal. Her blood pressure never decreased <110 mm Hg, and there were no situations seemingly causing acute tubular necrosis to account for deterioration in renal function. She required ventilatory support for worsening breathlessness. She could not be weaned off the ventilator and persisted in renal failure requiring dialysis. The left ventricular function was normal, and she did not need any inotropes. There was mild diastolic dysfunction only. The right ventricular size and function were normal. There were no signs of sepsis. After a few dialyses, a cardiac test was done that revealed the cause of her problems.

Can you guess the diagnosis?

Pause and think before you click the answer:

Answer: The physician in charge realized the dynamic afterload dependence of MR. With the control of her BP, MR had improved significantly. However, the onset of renal failure as the BP was lowered was suspicious of renal artery stenosis even though the Doppler was normal. A CT angio done revealed a totally unsuspected picture. Can you decipher the CT angio (**Video 3** and **Fig. 2**). Please see the video before seeing the figure and find the answer.

Video 3

Answer:

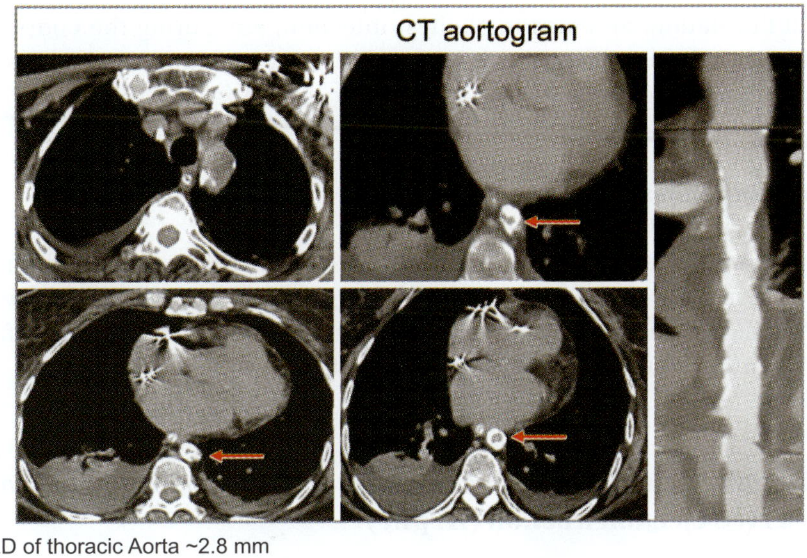

Fig. 2: Computed tomography (CT) angio pictures.
Courtesy: Dr Manoj @SRM Chennai.

She had severe calcification in a very tortuous aorta causing an acquired coarctation (Coral Reef Aorta) **(Fig. 3)**. Since the CART was done through right radial artery, this obstruction was not apparent then. The femoral pulses were not palpated by physicians in an elderly lady. After a very difficult intervention involving several balloon dilatations of the aorta, some decrease in aortic gradient was obtained and her renal failure improved. She was discharged home in a stable condition.

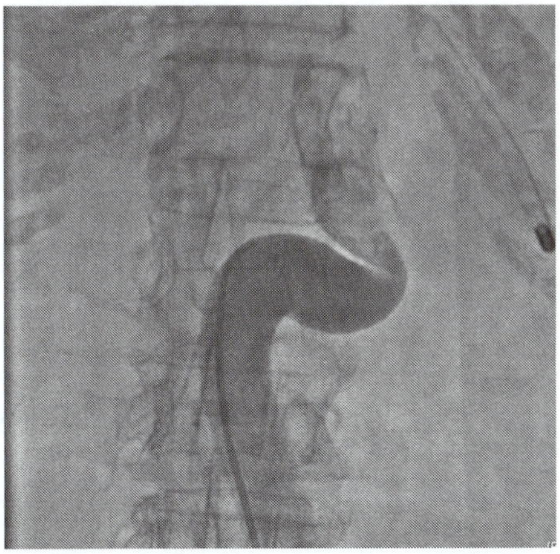

Fig. 3: Aortic angiogram showing tortuous aorta. The calcification and narrowing are better seen on the computed tomography (CT) angiogram **(video)**.

Although viewing it this way makes the diagnosis quite easy, this story is simplified for the sake of convenience [as she had gastrointestinal (GI) bleed, atrial fibrillation, an episode of chest infection, etc. during the course of illness], but the persistence of the treating physician in pursuing the missing link is remarkable.

Learning points:

- Mitral regurgitation is load dependent.
- Acquired coarctation may happen due to aortic calcification and might be severe.
- Intelligent pursuit of an unexplained phenomenon in a patient is often rewarding, but discrimination is required.

Sidelight: What are the mechanisms of MR in heart failure with preserved ejection fraction (HFpEF)?

(*Sidelights are food for thought—provided to increase your curiosity:* So as a rule, do not read these answers before you try to answer them yourself. The answers provided here are not intended to be exhaustive.)

Answer: MR in the absence of valvar pathology results from imbalance of tethering forces and contracting forces. In HFpEF, moderate to severe MR has been reported in 3–30% of patients. The reasons could be many including atrial myopathy, annular dilatation, subclinical ventricular dysfunction, increased left ventricular end-diastolic pressure (LVEDP) and LA pressures resisting the closure, regional myocardial dysfunction influencing tethering, etc. It is considered a poor prognostic marker.

CASE

22

Paroxysmal Hypertension in an Elderly Lady

"Knowledge is that, which liberates."

—Vishnu Puran

A 62-year-old diabetic lady reported to emergency services with atypical chest pain, breathlessness, and hypertension. 2 weeks earlier, she was admitted to a local facility with similar complaints and was diagnosed as having hypertensive urgency. She was not known to have hypertension earlier. She was treated with amlodipine, losartan, hydrochlorothiazide, metoprolol, and sertraline [a selective serotonergic reuptake inhibitor (SSRI)] with moderate blood pressure control. However, 4 days before presenting to us, she had another episode of severe hypertension with disorientation. Magnetic resonance imaging (MRI) brain was normal. She was treated with the addition of intravenous mannitol and furosemide to the antihypertensive drugs and was transferred to this emergency facility. Other details were not available.

On presentation, she was conscious, in distress, and confused. Her heart rate was 65 beats/min, blood pressure was 160/117 mm Hg, and chest auscultation showed isolated crackles and few rhonchi. Her ECG **(Fig. 1A)** showed ST-T changes with QT prolongation, and the chest X-ray showed increased bronchovascular markings with mild pulmonary venous hypertension **(Fig. 2)**. The trop I was negative and saturation was 88%. She was treated with Bi-PAP support and intravenous nitroglycerine and oral antihypertensives. Her serum sodium was 110 mEq/L, and serum potassium was 2.6 mEq/L. The blood sugar, liver function test, renal function test, and thyroid function tests were within normal limits. The echocardiogram showed normal left ventricular function and mild left ventricular hypertrophy.

(The format of this case is different from the previous cases, as there are many learning points. You may pause before all the bold type font and consider the possibilities before reading further).

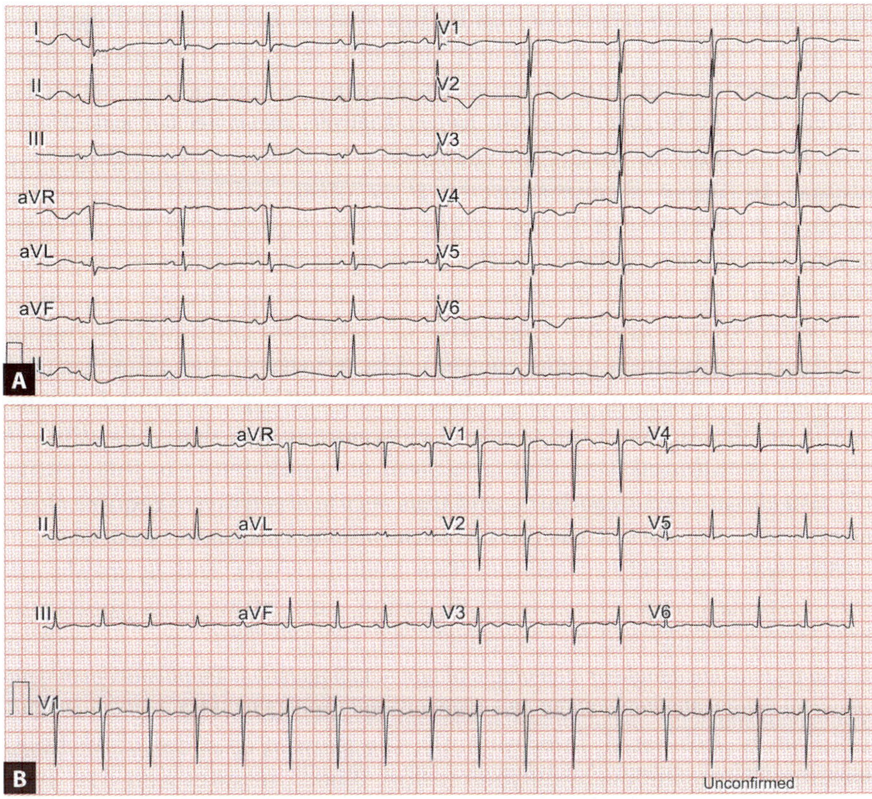

Figs. 1A and B: (A) ECG at presentation showing widespread ST-T changes and a QT interval of 500 ms; (B) ECG after correction of electrolyte abnormality within normal limits.

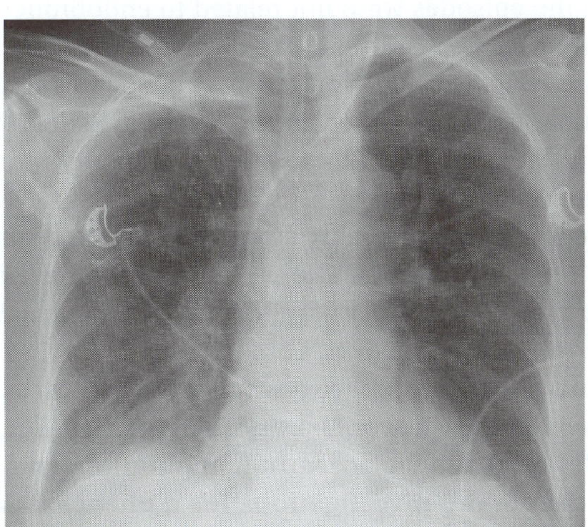

Fig. 2: Chest X-ray showed increased bronchovascular markings with mild pulmonary venous hypertension.

Hypertension with hypokalemia brings several differential diagnoses to mind. However, in an elderly diabetic lady with atypical chest pain, hypertension and dyspnea presenting to emergency services, myocardial ischemia, and/or heart failure need to be ruled out first. Hypertension might be secondary to ischemia or pulmonary edema; in these circumstances, it is often difficult to identify whether hypertension is the cause or consequence of myocardial ischemia or heart failure. In the present case, findings of negative trop I, normal echocardiogram, and ECG showing changes typical of dyselectrolytemia are not suggestive of ischemia. (Although ischemia and dyselectrolytemia might coexist). The priority in her management is to treat severe hyponatremia, hypokalemia, and hypertension. Extreme care is needed to avoid the cerebral consequences of demyelination. It might be mentioned here that treatment of hypokalemia in this setting will also elevate serum sodium, and thus serum electrolytes require close monitoring. The chest X-ray did not show obvious pulmonary edema.

She was electively intubated. The hyponatremia and hypokalemia were corrected over 3 days with 3% saline, and intravenous potassium replacement as advised by a nephrologist. Her pro-BNP was reported to be 218 pg/mL (normal for <75 years of age—125 pg/mL). The blood pressure was well controlled and ECG changes normalized **(Fig. 1B)**. However, she could not be extubated. Intermittently, she showed episodes of flushing, sweating, disorientation, and hypertension. Blood pressures were 170–190/90–100 mm Hg during these episodes. The monitor showed heart rates varying from 80–110 beats/min and saturations 95–96%. During those times, an endotracheal tube was well in position, the ventilatory settings were not altered and the episodes were not related to endobronchial suctioning. The blood sugar levels were normal. The daytime pressures otherwise were 120–130/70–80 mm Hg. The antihypertensive therapy was continued. During the hospitalization, there was an episode of chest infection that was treated with colistin and gentamycin. Biochemical parameters including serum electrolytes, serum calcium, phosphorus, and magnesium levels were normal **(Table 1)**. There was no history of hypertension, sudden death, or endocrine disorders in the patient's family. The patient did not have any significant medical history except the history of mild seasonal bronchial asthma in the last 3 years intermittently treated with bronchodilators.

Approach to a patient with paroxysmal hypertension may be difficult. Box 1 enumerates the causes of paroxysmal hypertension.

The episodes of headache, sweating, palpitation, and severe hypertension often dictate the investigations for a pheochromocytoma, but such a diagnosis is found in <2% of the patients in whom it is suspected. In fact, patients with pheochromocytoma do not typically have flushing, but they appear pale during the episodes. Hypertension and disproportionate

TABLE 1: Laboratory parameters of the patient.

Hemoglobin (g/dL)	13.6
TLC (/mm^3)	13,500
Platelet count (/mm^3)	42,800
Blood urea (mg/dL)	21.4
Creatinine (mg/dL)	0.65
Sodium (mEq/L)	137
Potassium (mEq/L)	4.2
Chloride (mEq/L)	97
Calcium (mg/dL)	8.4
Phosphorus (mg/dL)	3.7
Magnesium (mg/dL)	1.8
RBS (mg/dL)	138
CRP (mg/L)	1.4
Procalcitonin (ng/mL)	0.03
Troponin I	8.7
CPK MB (U/L)	38
CPK total (U/L)	43
NT-proBNP (pg/mL)	218
Bilirubin total (mg/dL)	0.5
ALT (U/L)	19
AST (U/L)	18
ALP (U/L)	109
Protein total (g/dL)	7.2
Albumin (g/dL)	4.2
Globulin (g/dL)	3
Plasma-free metanephrine (pg/mL)	10.3
24 hours urine VMA (mg/24 hours)	1
INR	1.01
APTT second	42.8
HbA1c	9%

(ALP: alkaline phosphatase; ALT: alanine aminotransferase; APTT: activated partial thromboplastin time; AST: aspartate aminotransferase; CPK-MB: creatine phosphokinase-MB; CRP: C-reactive protein; INR: international normalized ratio; HbA1c: hemoglobin A1c; RBS: random blood sugar; TLC: total leukocyte count; VMA: vanillylmandelic acid)

BOX 1: Causes of paroxysmal hypertension.

- Secondary to sympathetic drive in patients with myocardial ischemia, hypoglycemia, or respiratory insufficiency
- *Classic causes:*
  - Pheochromocytoma
  - Drugs and toxins
  - Clonidine withdrawal
  - Erratic antihypertensive treatment
  - Binge drinking
  - Labile hypertension
  - Renal artery stenosis* and adrenal adenoma*
  - Neurogenic hypertension
  - Autonomic seizures
  - Panic attacks
  - Rare systemic illnesses such as carcinoid syndrome,† systemic porphyria, and systemic mastocytosis†

*Typically present with resistant hypertension, but rarely may present with paroxysms.
†Commonly hypotension, but rarely may present with hypertension.

hypokalemia (in this case possibly induced by overzealous diuretic use) might suggest a hyperreninemic state. Hyperaldosteronism and renal artery stenosis should be excluded. These disorders are generally considered in patients with resistant hypertension, but rarely they might cause paroxysmal hypertension. Variations in the autonomic state of the individual might conceivably cause the paroxysm in these conditions although no systematic studies are available regarding the paroxysmal nature of hypertension in renal artery stenosis or adrenal adenoma.

Labile hypertension and paroxysmal hypertension may be difficult to distinguish. Although fluctuations of blood pressures in patients with essential hypertension are of the order of 25 mm Hg, but the fluctuations might be more in the elderly. The presence of distinct symptomatic episodes with distress makes labile hypertension less likely.

The patient underwent a series of tests to uncover the cause of paroxysmal hypertension. The abdominal ultrasound showed normal-sized kidneys and both the renal arteries were had normal Doppler wave forms. A 24-hour urinary vanillylmandelic acid (VMA) was 10.3 mg (normal—<13.2 mg), and plasma metanephrine (58 pg/mL—normal values—<65 pg/mL) was normal. The abdominal contrast-enhanced computed tomography (CECT) **(Fig. 3)** did not reveal any mass, lymphadenopathy, or any significant abnormality. Colonic diverticula were noted. Both the adrenals were normal. The CECT chest **(Fig. 4)** was also done and showed minor pulmonary emboli not accounting for symptoms. There were no paraganglioma. The venous Doppler of lower limbs was normal. She had a normal MRI and a normal carotid artery Doppler. The tests for carcinoid syndrome were not available, and the diagnosis was considered unlikely. There was no suspicion of the use of illicit drugs or toxin ingestion. The aldosterone and renin profiling were not pursued further as the imaging studies were normal and electrolytes remained normal after initial stabilization.

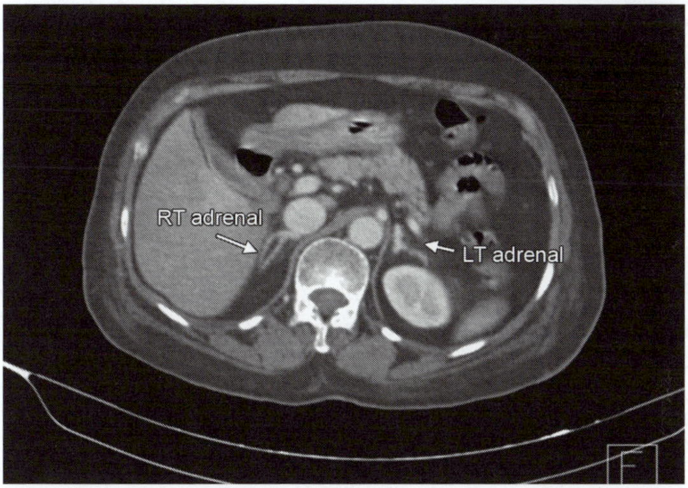

Fig. 3: Axial contrast CT abdomen image showing normal adrenals.

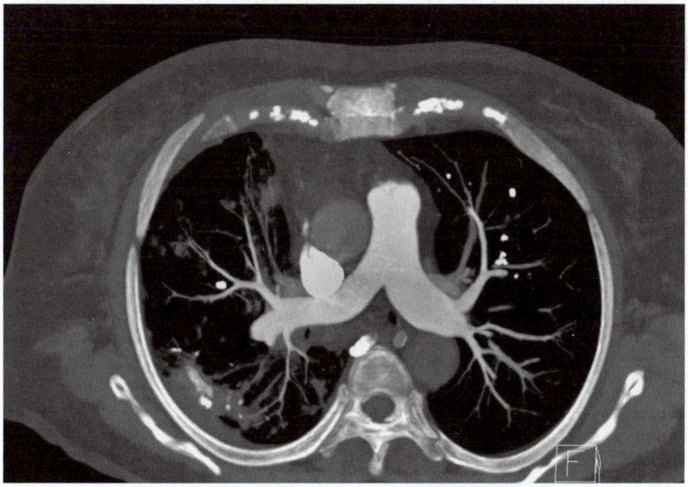

Fig. 4: Maximal intensity projection axial CT pulmonary angiography.

What would you consider?

The consideration for unusual causes of paroxysmal hypertension such as pseudopheochromocytoma is warranted. Often these patients have a traumatic stress disorder in the past, and they mount a hypertensive response to any stressor—psychological or physical. This patient was on SSRI although there was no past history of any major psychiatric illness or stress disorder. Alternatively, other causes of neurogenic hypertension such as autonomic seizures should also be considered. There is no evidence of any drug ingestion or toxins. Sometimes, the episodes of paroxysms of hypertension might be due to systemic illness such as systemic mastocytosis or porphyria. It is often reasonable to revisit the entire story for missing links when faced with a clinical dilemma.

The tendon reflexes were normal. There were no abnormal movements, eyeball uprolling, or myoclonic jerks during the episodes. The patient was planned for an EEG. However, during one of the episodes, when we were transiently able to extubate her, it appeared that the patient had difficulty keeping the eyes open **(Video 1)**.

Video 1

On questioning the caregiver, he reported that for the last 2 months, she could not keep her eyes open when the blood pressure was high. This story, coupled with the raised dome of the diaphragm on a subsequent X-ray **(Fig. 5)** initiated the consideration of reactionary hypertension to any respiratory difficulties.

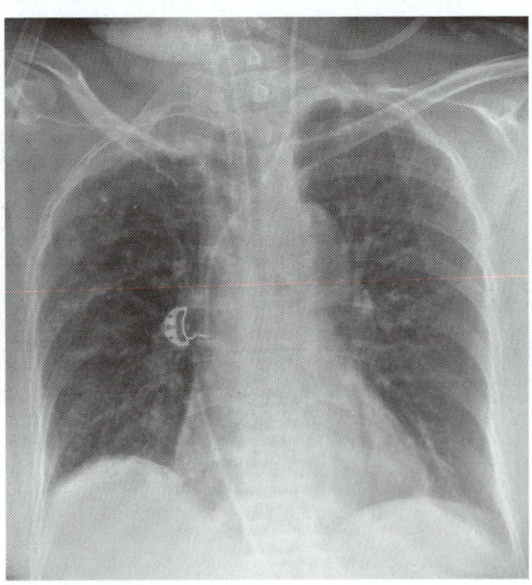

Fig. 5: A subsequent chest X-ray during the clinical course showing a mildly elevated right dome of the diaphragm.

The arterial blood gases twice during the episodes showed partial pressure of carbon dioxide (PCO_2) of 70 and 75 mm and increased alveolar arterial gradient for oxygen. The arterial blood gases at other times were within normal range. The test for acetylcholine receptor antibodies for myasthenia gravis was strongly positive. (Patient—8 nmol/L, normal values <0.4 nmol/L). She was shifted to a neurology facility for further management, but unfortunately, she succumbed to her illness shortly thereafter with sepsis and multiorgan failure.

Discussion

The final diagnosis in this patient was myasthenic crisis. Myasthenia crisis may rarely be the initial manifestation of myasthenia gravis. The diagnosis of myasthenia was entirely missed, and the patient was labeled as a case of hypertensive encephalopathy initially. All the later evaluation was targeted at unraveling the cause of the paroxysm of hypertension. What alterations were precisely used to trigger the crisis while the patient was on a ventilator remains unclear. Diuretic-induced hypokalemia initially and antibiotics and other drugs used subsequently in the management of the patient could have worsened the myasthenic weakness. The lack of hypoxia on a monitor during the episodes was related to the high fraction of inspired oxygen (FiO_2) that she was receiving. Arterial blood gas analysis during the episodes was not considered in the absence of hypoxia on the monitor. Once the clinical context was realized, the arterial blood gas did show CO_2 retention during the episodes.

Hypertension secondarily to sympathetic overdrive due to hypoglycemia, myocardial ischemia, or respiratory insufficiency may masquerade as a hypertensive emergency, and the real illness may be missed. This case illustrates the value of clinical evaluation in the era of technology dependence. An earlier appraisal of her clinical story could have alerted to the correct cause of the paroxysms of hypertension, possibly sparing unnecessary investigations and prompting appropriate therapy. Unfortunately, this scenario is not uncommon nowadays, with physicians adhering more to the monitors than to the patient's faces. Thus raising the correct clinical context from clinical history and physical examination remains a central aspect of clinical decision making.

Learning points: Paroxysmal hypertension in a patient may result from numerous clinical conditions. Hypertension secondarily to sympathetic overdrive due to hypoglycemia, myocardial ischemia, or respiratory insufficiency may masquerade as a hypertensive emergency, and the real illness may be missed. Thus, raising the correct clinical context from clinical history and physical examination remains a central aspect of clinical decision making.

(*Source:* Kothari SS, Agarwal S, Sharma V. Paroxysmal Hypertension: A Grave Cause. J Assoc Physicians India. 2024;72(12):83-6.)

Sidelights: Since the case already has several sidelights in the discussion, no additional sidelights posted for this case.

CASE

23

Failure to Wean Off the Bypass in a Child

"When you have eliminated all which is impossible, then whatever remains, however improbable, must be the truth."

—Arthur Conan Doyle

A 6-month-old child had supracardiac total anomalous pulmonary venous connection (TAPVC) to the right superior vena cava (SVC) and heart failure. He had moderate pulmonary hypertension and normal biventricular function. He was operated under cardiopulmonary bypass (CPB). The operation was routine and was done by an experienced cardiac surgeon. After coming off the bypass, the vertical vein was ligated. After the ligation, the patient showed bradycardia and decreased contractions. The bypass was reinitiated. After stabilization, the attempt to come off the bypass was done, but again the sequence was repeated. It was observed by the experienced surgeon that the heart was becoming somewhat dusky. The routine intraoperative echocardiography did not pick up anything abnormal. The coronary arteries were normal. Can you guess what could be the problem?

Pause and think before you click the answer:

Answer: The heart was becoming dusky, and the coronary arteries were normal; therefore, a problem with coronary venous drainage was suspected. Preoperatively, there were no problems; thus, the operation must have altered something in the drainage. Coronary sinus atresia was suspected, and the right atrium was opened **(Fig. 1)**. The coronary sinus orifice was indistinct with a membrane obstructing it, rendering it effectively atretic. It was opened in the left atrium. Subsequently, the patient came off bypass without any problem and was discharged home. Postoperatively, the coronary venous return would be draining to the left atrium that might cause minimal but clinically undetectable desaturation.

In clinical decision making, it is the context generation which is the most important step. A context of normal ventricles preop, a routine surgery, and a postoperative dusky heart; if looked at like this leaves no other diagnosis except some problem with cardiac ischemia—and thereafter even a rare entity like this seems inevitable! Coronary sinus atresia is a rare anomaly. It might be missed during echocardiography.

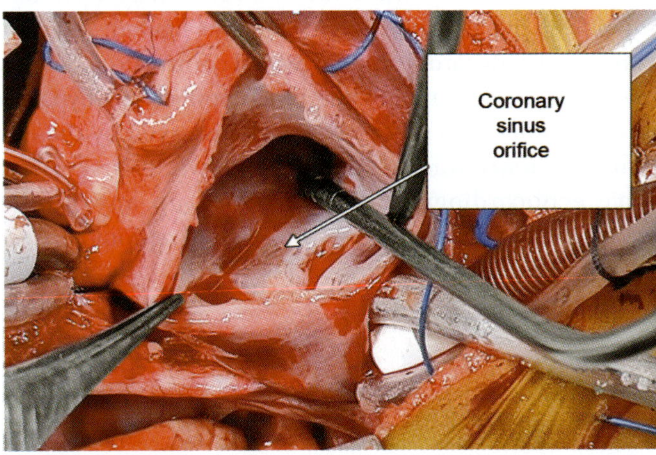

Fig. 1: Intraoperative picture showing coronary sinus atresia.

(*Source:* Dhanak R, Halder V, Shah R, Mishra A, Kothari SS. Failure to wean off after a routine total anomalous pulmonary venous connection operation: An uncommon association. Ann Pediatr Cardiol. 2023;16(5):367-9.)

Learning points: Undiagnosed coronary sinus atresia may sometimes be a cause of postoperative problems. Failure to wean off the CPB circuit could be from a number of causes, but we must think physiologically as to what has been altered by the operation, and then try to investigate in the context of that situation. Coronary sinus atresia unmasked due to left superior vena cava (LSVC) ligation followed by cardiac dysfunction has been more commonly recognized.

Sidelights:

1. **What might be a cause of a similar problem of deterioration in left ventricular (LV) function after closing a nonrestrictive ventricular septal defect (VSD) or a patent ductus arteriosus (PDA)?**
2. **Sudden deterioration in LV function after an atrial septal defect (ASD) device closure?**

(*Sidelights are food for thought—provided to increase your curiosity:* So as a rule, do not read these answers before you try to answer them yourself. The answers provided here are not intended to be exhaustive.)

Answer: If there is no obvious cause, one might look for the left coronary artery from the pulmonary artery (LCAPA) as the PA pressures reduce after the closure and the ischemia might manifest which was not there earlier because the coronary was perfused antegradely from PA and could have been missed. Such cases have been published!

- An aberrant circumflex artery from the right coronary sinus might get compressed by the ASD device. This anatomy should be checked on echo prior to the device closure in an ASD patient. Not all the patients with anomalous circumflex artery get the compression, so a refined judgment is needed, but it is important to be aware of the entity.

CASE

24

Cyanosis in a Newborn with Normal Heart

"From Wonder into Wonder, Existence Opens".

—Lao Tzu

An 8-day-old newborn was referred for evaluation of cyanosis and distress. His oximeter showed 75% saturation in the right upper limb. There was significant cardiomegaly, heart rate (HR) of 130 beats/min, and a brisk pulse with a BP of 90/50 mm Hg. The echo did not show any structural defect except moderate atrial septal defect (ASD). There was right-to-left shunting through the ASD. The estimated pulmonary artery systolic pressure from tricuspid regurgitation jet was 70 mm Hg. The clinical diagnosis considered by some was persistent pulmonary hypertension of newborn (PPHN). The X-ray is overpenetrated but shows significant cardiomegaly **(Fig. 1)**. There was no meconium aspiration or clinical likelihood of a pulmonary problem.

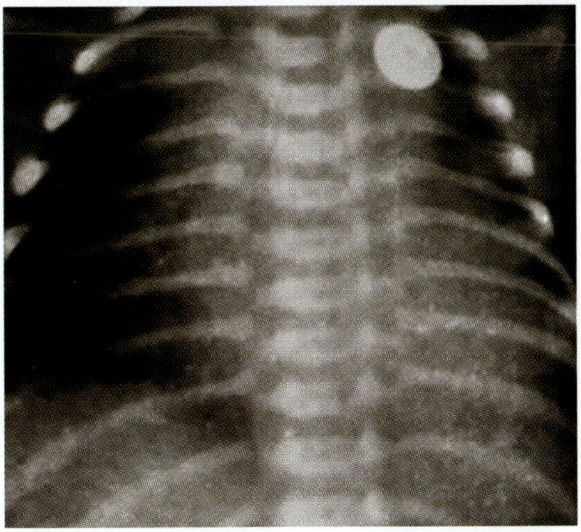

Fig. 1: Chest X-ray showing significant cardiomegaly.

The echo showed a structurally normal heart. In view of the clinical findings, the echo was repeated.

What would you think it could show?

Pause and think before you click the answer:

Answer: The repeat echo of the suprasternal view is shown here **(Video 1)**.

Video 1

What is the diagnosis?
Can you enumerate the causes of this finding? (See learning points). What could be the diagnosis of this child?

Answer: Because the child was blue, one does not consider systemic arteriovenous (AV) fistula easily. But with a patent foramen ovale (PFO)/ ASD in a newborn, increased venous return from AV fistula causes a right to left shunt and cyanosis that may confuse the clinical picture. Finally, the patient was found to have an aneurysm of the vein of Galen malformation. The brisk pulses in the wake of severe pulmonary arterial hypertension were not in favor of persistent pulmonary hypertension (PPHN). Hence, an echo was repeated that showed aortic flow reversal in the arch and high flow in the superior vena cava (SVC). Retrospectively, a loud hum was also auscultated on the cranium of the neonate. (Caution: A faint hum may normally be heard on the cranium in neonates.)

The carotid angio shows the massive vein of Galen malformation **(Fig. 2)**.

The cranial ultrasound from another patient showing a vein of Galen malformation (**Video 2**).

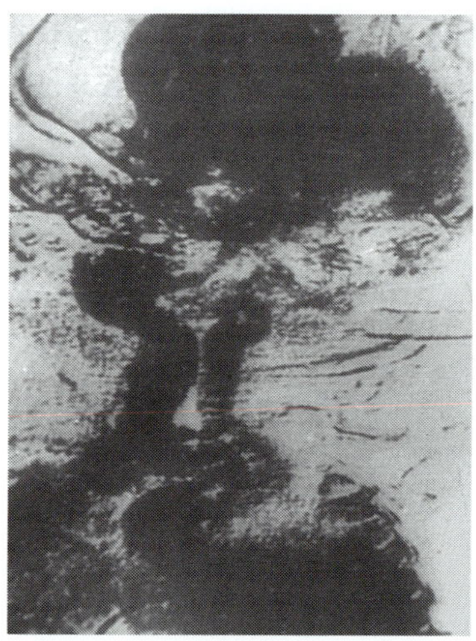

Fig. 2: Vein of Galen malformation on carotid angiogram (DSA).

Video 2

Learning points: Causes of aortic flow reversal to be considered—Aortic regurgitation, Truncal regurgitation, hemitruncus, coronary AV fistula, systemic to PA collaterals from the upper body, systemic AV fistula-like vein of Galen malformation, ruptured sinus of Valsalva, and aortopulmonary window.

(Note that PDA and high flow states such as anemia do not cause significant aortic flow reversal in the arch).

Further, severe PAH with compromised left ventricular output can cause flow reversal in the arch as in hypoplastic left heart syndrome (HLHS), or severe aortic stenosis with PDA.

Sidelights: Can aortic flow reversal be intermittent?

Severe hypercarbia or hypoxia may possibly cause intermittent flow reversal (because of cerebral vasodilatation). See **Video 3** of a neonate with TGA showing no flow reversal during sedated state, but shows flow reversal during crying in **Video 4**.

Video 3 **Video 4**

(*Source:* Kothari SS, Pathak NL, Banerji N, Champaneri B. Intermittent flow reversal in the aortic arch. Ann Pediatr Cardiol. 2023;16(5):385-6.)

- Another case of brisk pulses and heart failure with normal structure in an infant:

  A 1-year-old infant with poor feeding, respiratory distress, and cardiomegaly. His X-ray is shown in **Figure 3** (poor film).

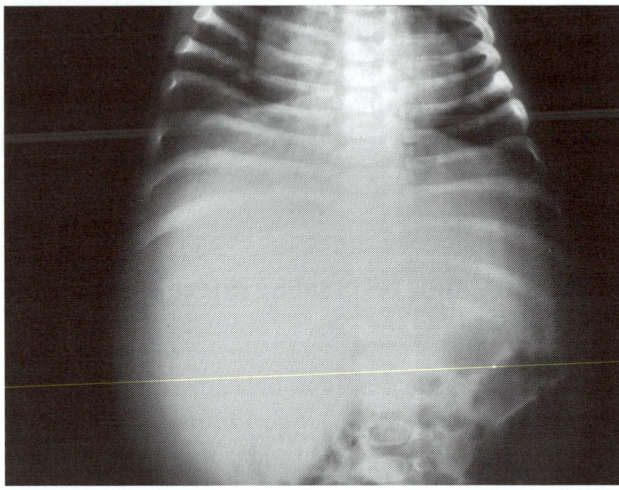

Fig. 3: Chest X-ray (poor film).

He had no anemia, brisk pulses, and normal cardiac echo except for biventricular dilatation and normal contractility. Thus, a setting for high-output heart failure appears likely. The liver ultrasound is shown in **Figure 4**.

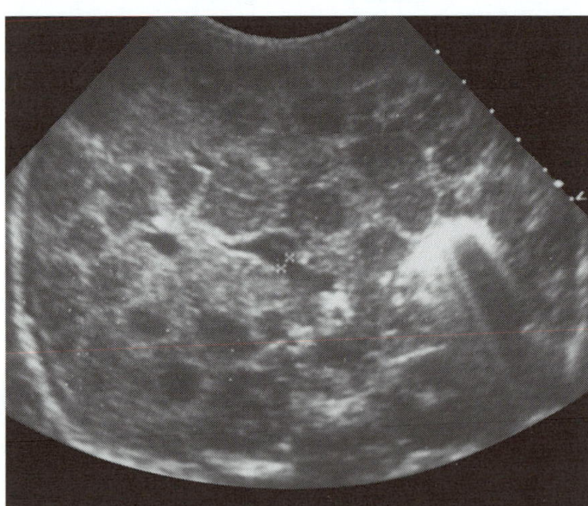

Fig. 4: Liver ultrasound.

Thus, he had hepatic hemangioendothelioma, a rare cause of high-output heart failure in infants. This is physiologically akin to hepatic arteriovenous fistula, usually a benign disease, and responds to hepatic artery embolization. Rarely, it may be malignant and metastasize. He responded to hepatic artery embolization. The disease is not well understood, and multiple therapeutic options are recommended; thus, it should be treated by a team of specialists.

Sidelights: Can you think of another cause of reversible PAH and brisk pulses in infants with no structural heart defect?

Video 5 **Video 6**

(*Courtesy:* Dr MK Usha & Dr Jay Rang nath; Sri Jayadeva Inst. Bangalore.)

These videos show an infant with brisk pulses and severe PAH before (**Video 5**), and *after* some treatment (**Video 6**).

Can you guess what could that be?

(*Sidelights are food for thought—provided to increase your curiosity:* So as a rule, do not read these answers before you try to answer them yourself. The answers provided here are not intended to be exhaustive.)

Answer: Infants in some parts of India in Karnataka, Kashmir, West Bengal, and other areas of the world where the babies have been fed exclusively on breast milk of malnourished mothers have severe thiamine deficiency. Curiously, they clinically may present with severe PAH as shown in the videos. Of course, when it is late in the clinical course, these infants present in shock and feeble pulses. A history of weak cries is typical of beriberi in infants! They improve rapidly with thiamine. The diagnosis may be completely missed unless one is aware of the possibility. Hence, palpating the pulse still remains useful!

CASE

25

Ventricular Aneurysms

"Uninterrupted practice of discrimination (between real and unreal) is the means to cessation of ignorance."

—Patanjali

A 26-year-old man presented with dull aching left-sided chest pain and progressive dyspnea of 2 months duration. The illness was subacute in onset and progressed significantly over 2 months duration. He was breathless on minimal exertion, but the chest pain was not related to exertion. On examination, he was thin built (BMI: 17 kg/m^2) and had mild pallor. The heart rate was 97 beats/min, respiratory rate was 24 breaths/min, and oxygen saturation was 99% on room air. Both upper limb pulses were feeble compared to the lower limb with significant difference in blood pressure (Rt arm: 80/60 mm Hg; Lt arm: 84/48 mm Hg; Rt ankle: 123/64 mm Hg, Lt ankle: 115/67 mm Hg). There was no carotid tenderness or a vascular bruit anywhere. On cardiovascular examination, a dyskinetic cardiac impulse was felt in the 6th intercostal space lateral to the midclavicular line in addition to the apical impulse. Heart sounds were normal with no murmur. After the examination, on probing, there was no history of trauma to the chest, nor any history of fever, constitutional symptoms, weight loss, or limb claudication. There was no significant past medical or family history. His laboratory parameters showed mild normocytic normochromic anemia (Hb: 9.6 g/dL), raised inflammatory markers (ESR: 55 mm, CRP: 116 mg/L), and normal renal and liver function tests. His chest X-ray and ECG are shown in **Figures 1 and 2**. The echo is shown in **Video 1** and **Figure 3**.

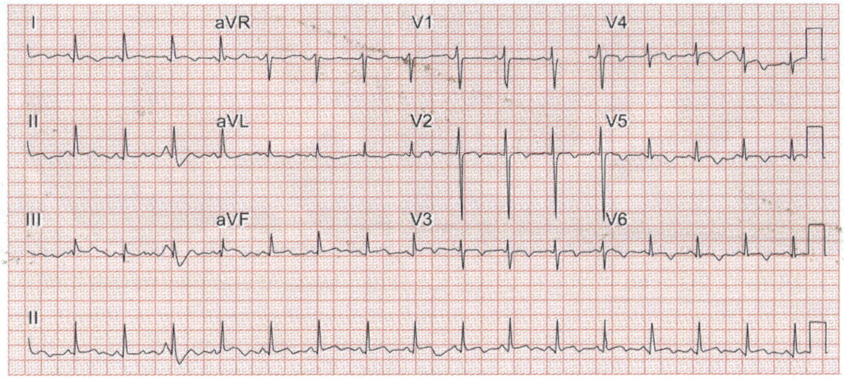

Fig. 1: ECG.

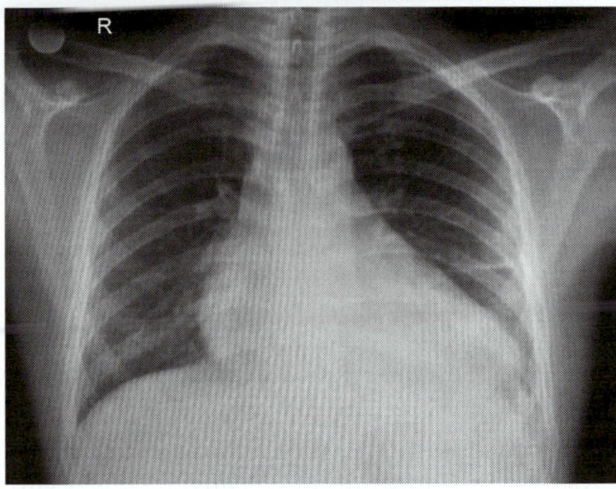

Fig. 2: Chest X-ray.

Video 1 **Video 2**

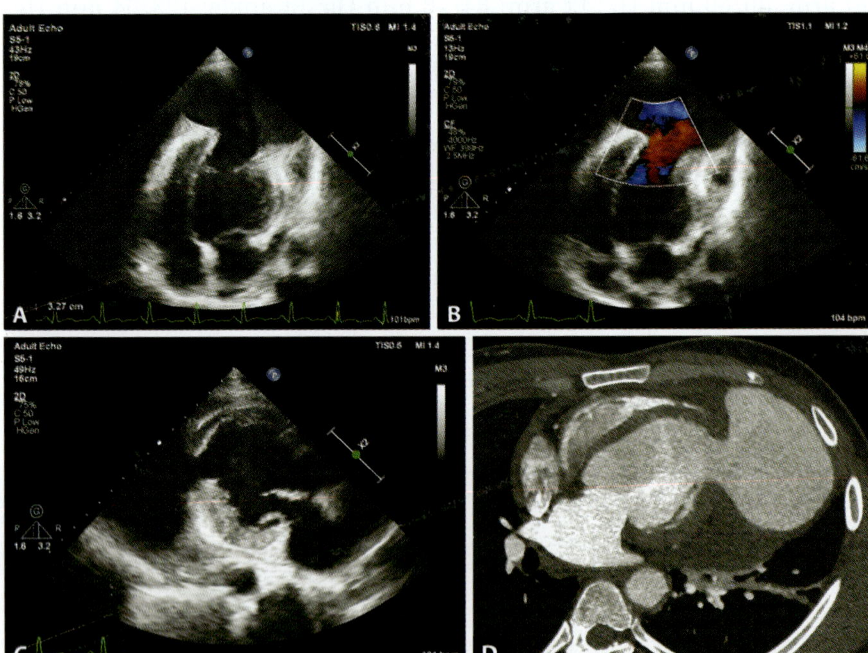

Figs. 3A to D: 2D echo image in apical four chambers (A) and parasternal long axis (B) view showing punched-out defect in left ventricular apex with a communicating large pseudoaneurysm. Doppler echo (C) showed unobstructed bidirectional flow between the left ventricle and pseudoaneurysm. Contrast-enhanced CT image (D) demonstrating large left ventricular pseudoaneurysm.

What is the etiology of the aneurysm?

Pause and think before you click the answer:

Answer: This patient had no history of trauma, ESR 55 mm Hg, and weak upper limb pulses. The computed tomography (CT) showed evidence of Takayasu aortoarteritis (**Figs. 4A to C**) with no coronary artery involvement. Ventricular aneurysms in Takayasu aortitis are rarely described and might result from coronary artery involvement and MI, or from myocarditis, or inflammation from the surrounding lymph nodes. The CT image is shown here.

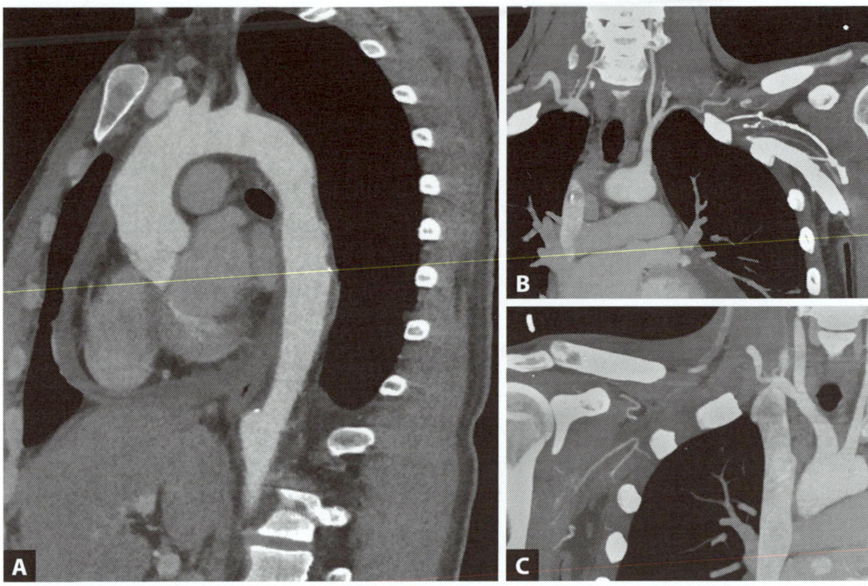

Figs. 4A to C: Contrast-enhanced arterial phase CT images show diffuse circumferential thickening of ascending whole aorta with its branches (A) and occlusion of bilateral subclavian arteries (B and C) with distal reformation with collaterals.

The aneurysm was resected surgically.

- A 6-year-old boy developed worsening fever and septic shock from staphylococcal septicemia. He recovered with antibiotics, and intensive care after a prolonged hospital course. During the illness, he had mild pericardial effusion also. A repeat echo after recovery is shown here **(Videos 3 to 5)**.

Video 3 Video 4 Video 5

What do these echo show?

Answer: There is a typical pseudoaneurysm of LV following an infective illness.

The CT images show the extensive pseudo aneurysm **(Figs. 5 and 6)**.

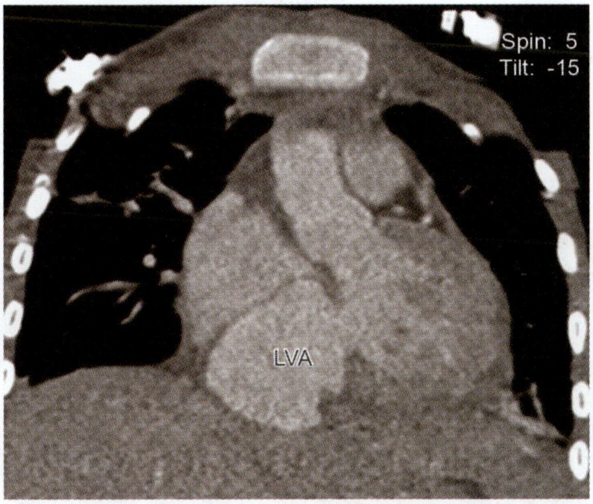

Fig. 5: Coronal computed tomography (CT) image showing LV pseudoaneurysm (LVA).

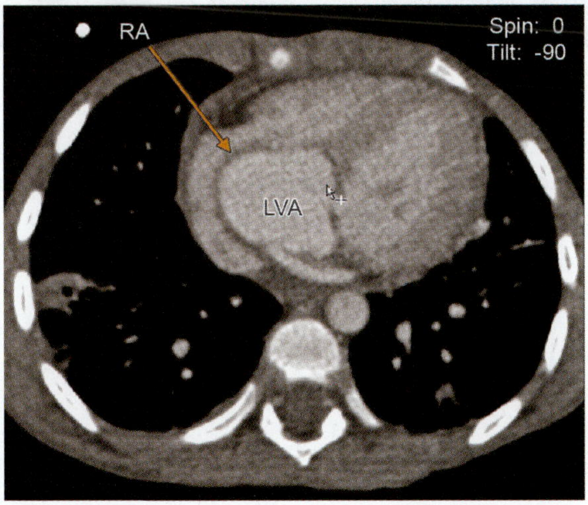

Fig. 6: Axial computed tomography (CT) image showing LV pseudoaneurysm compressing the right atrium (RA).

The pseudo aneurysm was repaired surgically.

(*Source:* Nair VV, Malankar D, Kothari SS, Das S, Gulati GS, Airan B. Unusual left ventricular pseudoaneurysm in a child after disseminated bacterial infection. World J Pediatr Congenit Heart Surg. 2014;5(1):121-3.)

- Another 5-year child with fever and the angiogram shown here **(Video 5A)**.

Video 5A

This is a small pseudoaneurysm.
The underlying osteomyelitis causing the pseudoaneurysm (arrow) was not initially realized **(Fig. 7)**.

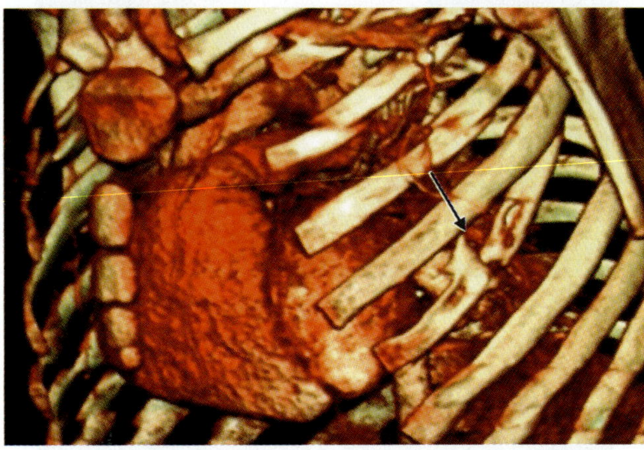

Fig. 7: Osteomyelitis causing pseudoaneurysm.

- A 45-year-old man had exertional angina for 1 year. He presented with acute retrosternal chest pain and sweating to the emergency. The ECG and chest X-ray are shown in **Figures. 8 and 9**.

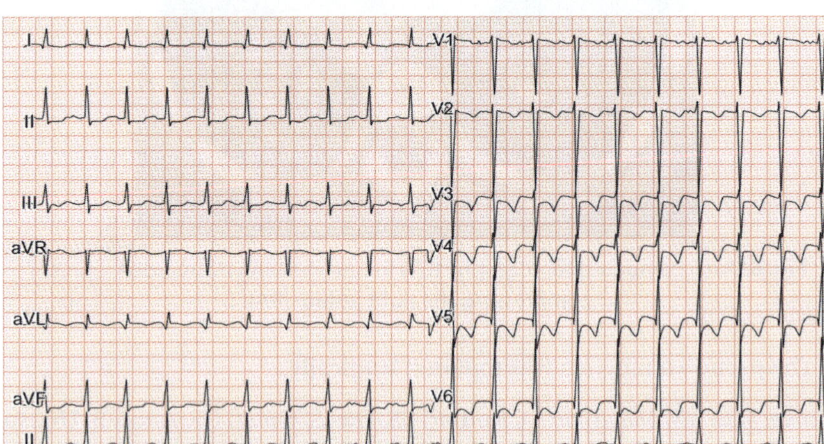

Fig. 8: ECG.

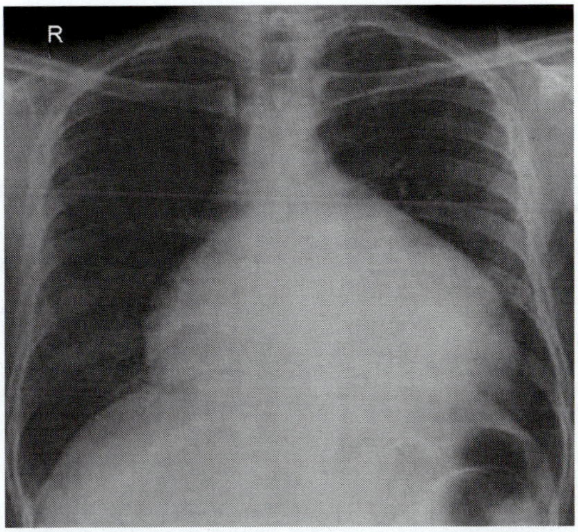

Fig. 9: Chest X-ray shows cardiomegaly.

The cardiac enzymes were normal. The echo showed mild left ventricular dysfunction with septal hypokinesia, but the subaortic area was very unusual **(Videos 6 to 9)**.

Video 6 Video 7 Video 8 Video 9

What do these echoes show?

Answer: A weird massive subaortic aneurysm extending anterosuperiorly is seen in the echo.

The CT shows the extent of the massive subaortic aneurysm that compresses the right pulmonary artery as well as coronary arteries **(Figs. 10A and B)**.

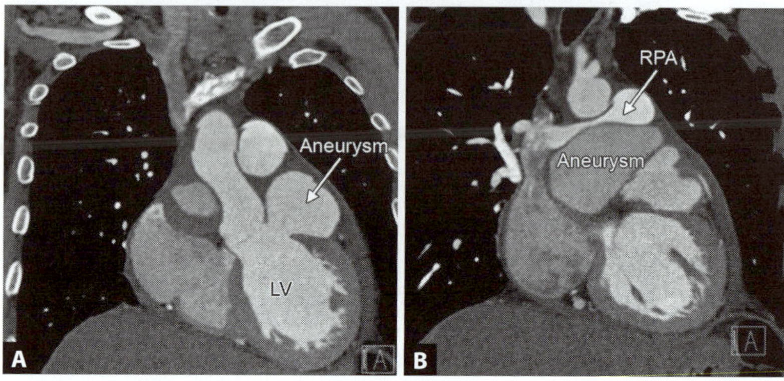

Figs. 10A and B: Subaortic aneurysm compressing right pulmonary artery.

The coronary arteries were stretched and compressed as seen on coronary angiogram images (**Figs. 11A to C**).

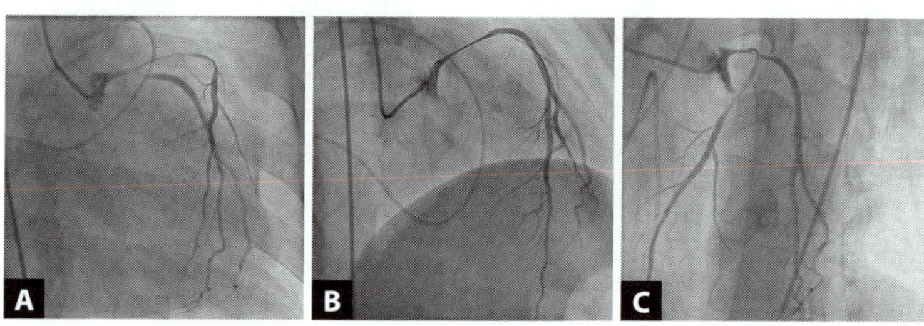

Figs. 11A to C: The left coronary artery angiogram images showing the stretching and compression of the left main coronary artery (LMCA) and mid part of the left anterior descending artery (LAD) as well as a proximal circumflex.

This was an idiopathic left ventricular subaortic aneurysm. The patient underwent aneurysmectomy under cardiopulmonary bypass.

Learning points: The ventricular aneurysms may occur from a variety of causes. Sometimes, they might produce surprising patterns. Takayasu aortoarteritis is a rare cause of ventricular aneurysm. Idiopathic subaortic aneurysms, though previously reported from Africa, are less well recognized. Such aneurysm may compress the coronary arteries and adjacent cardiac structures and may present with arrhythmia, ischemia, heart failure, or thromboembolism.

Sidelights:

1. **What is the difference between an aneurysm and a diverticulum?**
2. **What could cause the aneurysm shown in the first case (Fig. 3) in a patient in Brazil?**

(*Sidelights are food for thought—provided to increase your curiosity:* So as a rule, do not read these answers before you try to answer them yourself. The answers provided here are not intended to be exhaustive.)

Answer: The distinction of aneurysm, pseudoaneurysm, and diverticulum is generally simple. A pseudoaneurysm is a contained rupture, an aneurysm is an akinetic or dyskinetic part of protrusion that contains all the three layers of the heart, and diverticulum contracts with the ventricle and has all three layers. Sometimes a rare congenital LV diverticulum may pose a problem **(Video 10)**.

Video 10

(*Source:* Johnson JN, Pouraliakbar H, Mahdavi M, et al. Society for Cardiovascular Magnetic Resonance 2022 Cases of SCMR case series. J Cardiovasc Magn Reson. 2024 Summer;26(1):100007. doi: 10.1016/j.jocmr.2023.100007.)

Diverticulum can have a narrow neck and might sometimes get infarcted or fibrosis. Apical LV diverticulum with midline chest and abnormal defects are well recognized as Cantrell pentalogy.

- As to the patient from Brazil, a similar LV aneurysm has been seen in Chhaga's disease as well, though Takayasu aortitis also occurs in Brazil.

CASE

26

Lower Limb Deep Vein Thrombosis

"We read the world wrong and say that it deceives us."
—Rabindranath Tagore

A 28-year-old man had unprovoked left lower limb deep vein thrombosis (DVT) for which he was receiving acitrom 3 mg daily. His tests for thrombophilia were negative. A few months later, he had sudden onset breathlessness and chest discomfort while on oral anticoagulation medication. A computed tomography (CT) angio showed pulmonary embolism in both proximal pulmonary arteries **(Fig. 1)**. He was treated with heparin infusion and acitrom was changed to dabigatran at a local hospital.

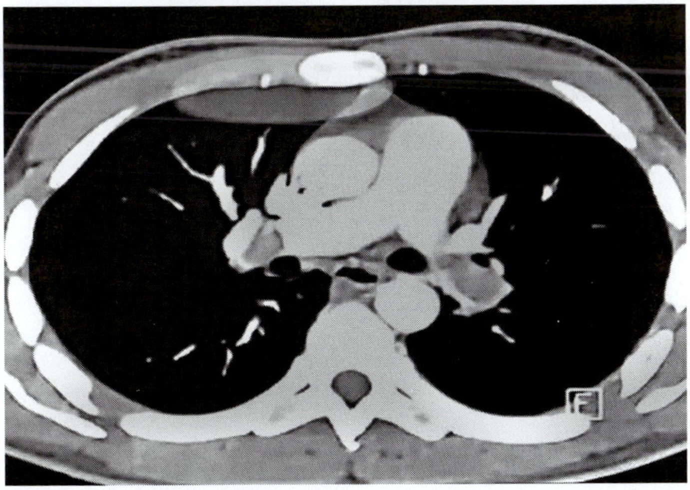

Fig. 1: Computed tomography (CT) angio showing thrombi in both pulmonary arteries.

The patient complained of thigh swelling for which a CT venogram was done that was reported to show extensive DVT and a large hematoma. The patient was receiving oral anticoagulants. The clinical picture is shown in **Figure 2**.

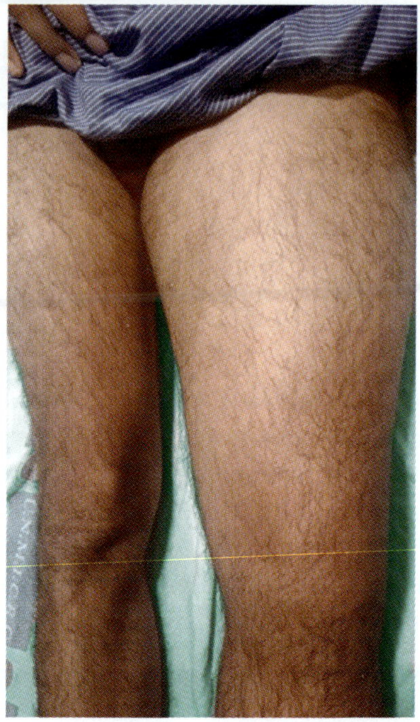

Fig. 2: Left thigh swelling while patient on anticoagulation.

What does this suggest? What should be done next? The clinician has made a terrible mistake.

Pause and think before you click the answer:

Answer: A repeat CT was done. The CT showed it was a large soft tissue mass (**Fig. 3**) misdiagnosed as hematoma that has metastasized to the pelvis and abdominal wall explaining his DVT and clinical course. The clinician unfortunately missed the therapeutic window for resection. The patient received chemotherapy. The picture shown is quite unlike a hematoma. Since soft tissue sarcoma is a rare tumor, this possibility is not commonly considered. A high index of suspicion for tumors in unprovoked DVT could have diagnosed the disease earlier. A tumor emboli and thrombus might be difficult to distinguish on imaging sometimes. The biopsy showed synovial sarcoma in this case.

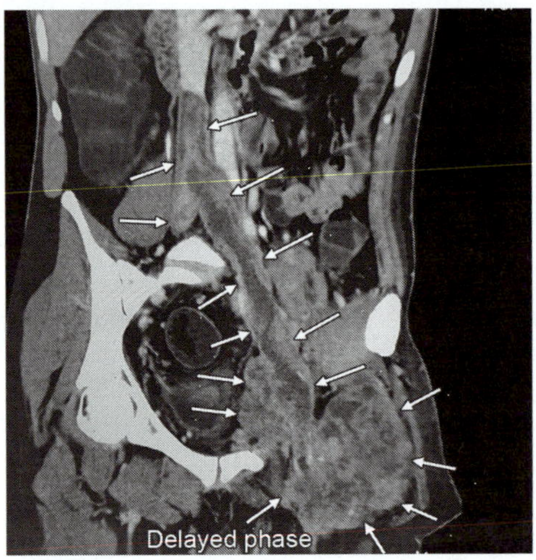

Fig. 3: Computed tomography (CT) showing the soft tissue mass and the venous thrombosis.

Learning points: Unprovoked DVT in a young should be viewed with suspicion. Although thrombophilia is the usual cause, fibrosarcoma and other rare soft tissue tumors may cause or masquerade as DVT.

Sidelights: Why left lower limb DVT is more common than right?

Answer: The answer is seen in the accompanying **Video 1**.

Video 1

The left common iliac vein is more horizontal and is prone to external compression from the right iliac artery and the fifth lumbar vertebra. This is known as May–Thurner syndrome. Video 1 is from a patient with May–Thurner syndrome. The anatomic predisposition is present in up to 20% of the population, whereas the May–Thurner syndrome is said to account for 2–5% of DVT cases. It is more common than generally believed. Of course, other factors of Virchow's triad causing DVT should always be considered: Recognition of May–Thurner syndrome is important to prevent the recurrences. It is more common in females, especially postpartum females.

Nutcracker syndrome is another vascular compression syndrome. Heard of it?

CASE

27

Lung Consolidation in a Post Mitral Valve Replacement Patient

"The art of knowing is knowing what to ignore".

—Rumi

A 44-year-old lady presented with low-grade fever and chills for a month and worsening dyspnea for the past 10 days. The patient had a cough and mild hemoptysis. She had mitral valve replacement (MVR) done with 27 mm St Jude's mechanical valve prosthesis for rheumatic mitral stenosis 3 years earlier. The patient had a closed mitral valvotomy (CMV) done 20 years earlier previously. On examination, she was febrile, had tachycardia 104 beats/min, and blood pressure of 110/70 mm Hg. Prosthetic valve sounds were normal and there was no murmur. There was bronchial breathing in the right chest posteriorly. Her chest X-ray is shown in **Figure 1**.

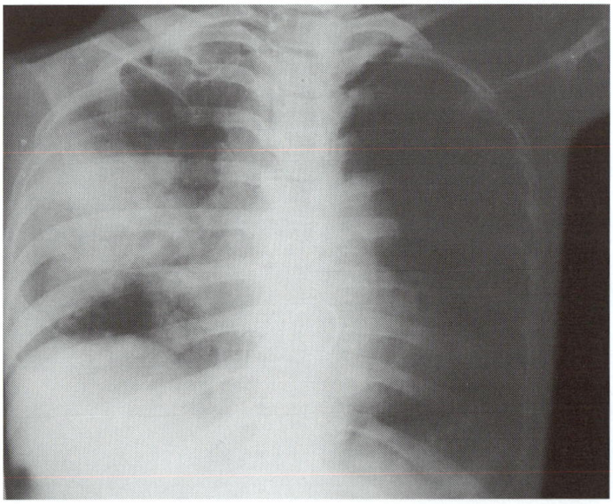

Fig. 1: Chest X-ray.

She had anemia (Hb 8 g%), TLC 11,000/mm^3, with 85% neutrophils, and raised ESR (58 mm in the first hour). There was mild proteinuria with serum creatinine of 2.4 mg%. The liver functions were normal. Blood cultures reported no growth. A computed tomography (CT) chest showed consolidation in the anterior segment of the right lower lobe, and bilateral nodular opacities with mediastinal lymph nodes. The bronchoscopy showed no mass, and the BAL showed acute inflammatory cells. The fine needle aspiration cytology (FNAC) from lymph nodes showed epitheloid granuloma but no acid-fast bacillus (AFB). A submandibular lymph node biopsy showed increased plasma cells but no caseating granuloma. The TTE showed a normally functioning prosthetic valve and an indistinct mass in the left atrium (LA). A TEE showed evidence of masses in the left and right atrium as shown in **Figures 2A and B**. The echo records are poor, but the masses in LA are well seen. The patient had an adequate INR on warfarin therapy, and LV function was normal.

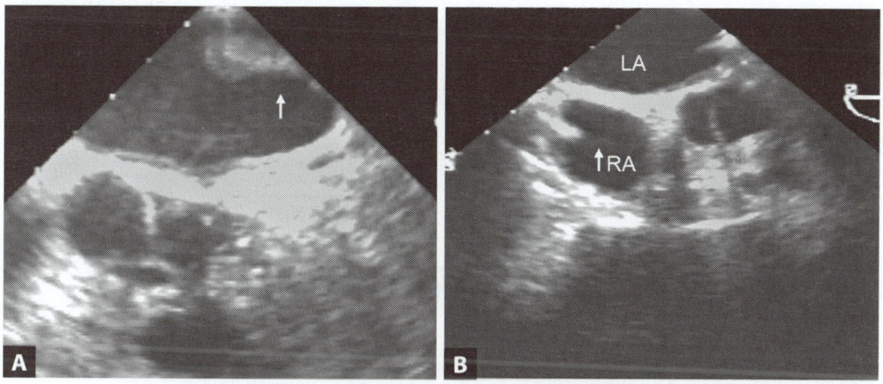

Figs. 2A and B: Transesophageal echocardiogram (TEE) showing mass in the left atrium (LA) (arrow) and in the right atrium (RA), respectively (arrow).

What may be the diagnosis?

Pause and think before you click the answer:

Answer: The patient did not improve on broad-spectrum antibiotics. While being investigated, she developed redness in the right eye from episcleritis. Her renal functions deteriorated, and chest X-ray remained the same. The antinuclear antibody (ANA) test was mildly positive, but cytoplasmic antineutrophil cytoplasmic antibody (cANCA) was strongly positive. On direct questioning (as often happens), she posited a history of a decrease in hearing and recurrent sinusitis-like illness in the past few months. Thus, the constellations of lung lesions, active sediments with renal involvement, and epitheloid granuloma with increased plasma cells with cANCA positive, and a cardiac mass led to the final diagnosis of Wegener's granulomatosis (now called granulomatous polyangiitis)!

(Unfortunately, she succumbed to the illness with worsening dyspnea and hemoptysis in the course of illness despite steroids and cyclophosphamide).

Learning points: Though infective endocarditis should always be considered for fever in post mitral valve replacement patients and remains a great mimic, a quicker appreciation of primary immunologic illness could have led to the earlier institution of appropriate therapy. Granulomatous polyangiitis or Wegener's granulomatosis may present with pericarditis (common), or may present with valvular involvement, and rarely as unusual masses.

Sidelights: An 18-year-old boy presented with a history of fever and dyspnoea for the last 2 weeks. He had congestive heart failure, severe MR, and mild AR on examination. The patient had no past history of rheumatic fever. He had anemia, ESR of 100 mm, and normal antistreptolysin O (ASLO) titers. The echo recordings are shown in Videos 1 and 2.

Video 1 Video 2

What is the diagnosis?

(*Sidelights are food for thought—provided to increase your curiosity:* So as a rule, do not read these answers before you try to answer them yourself. The answers provided here are not intended to be exhaustive.)

Answer: The picture is quite consistent with ARF as seen in the real world when ASLO is not always positive. A normal ASLO does not exclude acute rheumatic fever which is the most common cause of MR in a young adult in India. However, the valve morphology with thickening of leaflets and slight bulbous thickening at the aorto mitral junction was not very typical of RHD. The patient had recurrent aphthous ulcers (which is not uncommon in the population) and skin lesions are shown in **Figures 3A and B**. Further, he had mild proteinuria with a granular cast on urine examination (that might not be looked for routinely).

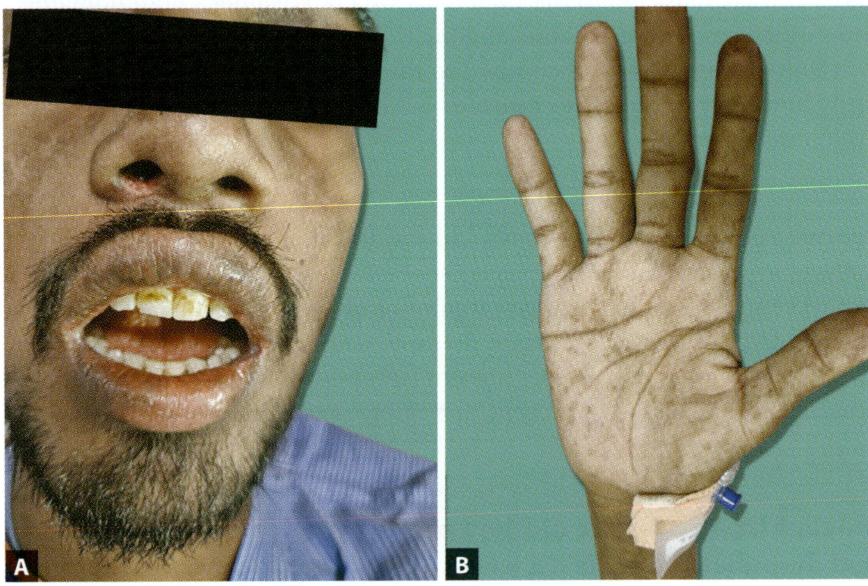

Figs. 3A and B: (A) Aphthous ulcers; (B) Healed skin lesions.

Aphthous ulcers alone are not enough to diagnose Behcet's disease. The patient did not have other features of Behcet's disease. His double-stranded DNA (dsDNA) was strongly positive (Sm+) and also the p-ANCA (MPO). The patient responded to steroids and immunosuppression with mycophenolate mofetil. A diagnosis of systemic lupus erythematosus (SLE)/mixed connective tissue disorder (MCTD) was made. A detailed discussion of vasculitis and cardiac disorders is not warranted here but suffices to think of vasculitis in appropriate settings. It is also important to remember that false positive ANA, or even ANCA might occur with infective endocarditis. Thus, as always, a comprehensive evaluation is the key to clinical diagnosis.

CASE

28

Cardiac Amyloidosis

"By our stumbling the world is perfected".

—Sri Aurobindo

A 55-year-old man had progressive breathlessness on exertion and abdominal distention of 3 months duration. He was in good health previously, but became quite symptomatic over the last 1 month. There was atypical chest pain on exertion. On examination, heart rate 100 beats/min, raised jugular venous pressure, and ascites were found. Cardiac auscultation was unremarkable. The Hb was 9 g, and ESR was 10 mm. The renal function tests were normal. Serum albumin and globulin were 3.1 and 2.2 g/dL, respectively (normal globulins 2.3–3.5 g/dL: gamma globulin fraction was reduced). The liver function tests were normal. The chest X-ray **(Fig. 1)** and ECG **(Fig. 2)** are shown here.

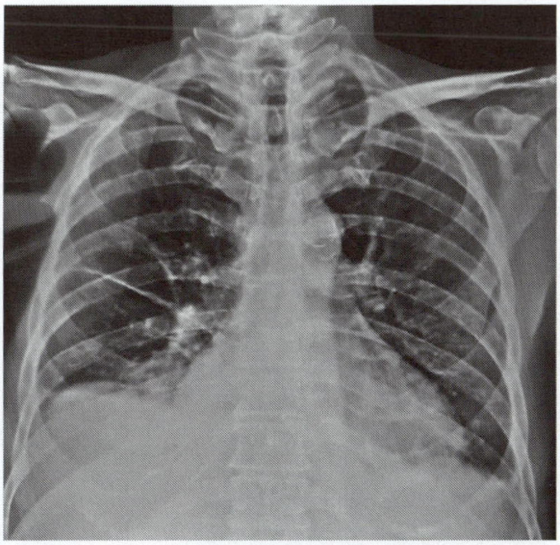

Fig. 1: Chest X-ray.

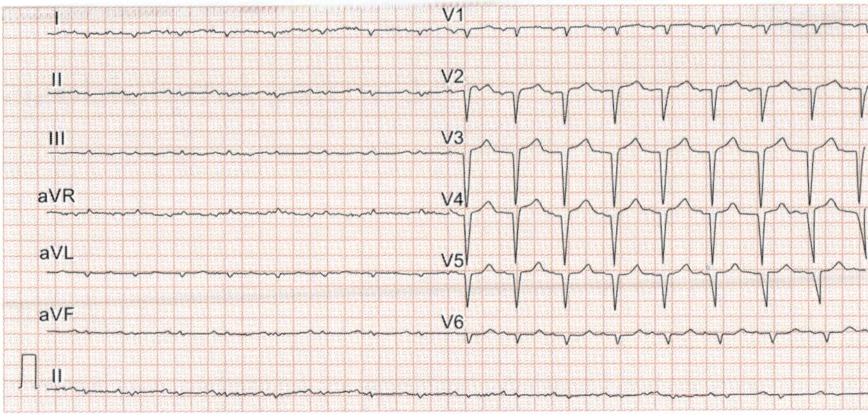

Fig. 2: ECG showing low voltages in limb leads.

The 2D echo is shown in **Videos 1 and 2**.

Video 1

Video 2

The tissue Doppler imaging (TDI) summary is shown in **Figure 3**.

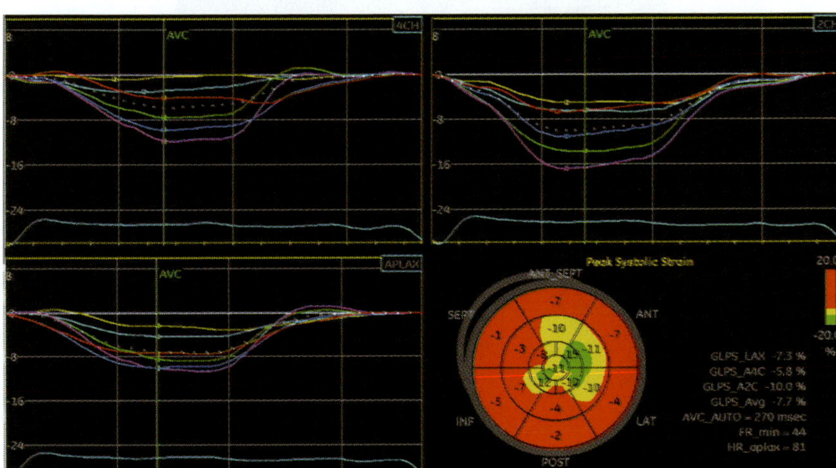

Fig. 3: Tissue Doppler image of amyloidosis patient showing a typical apical sparing of cardiac amyloidosis.

Thus a very typical pattern of amyloidosis seems to be present. Even the magnetic resonance imaging (MRI) done elsewhere showed subendocardial late gadolinium enhancement (LGE) that suggested amyloidosis.

However, no M band was seen on immunoelectrophoresis. Bence Jones proteins were not present. The bone marrow aspiration showed 5% plasma cells. Is this then transthyretin amyloidosis? What clinical features distinguish AL amyloid from transthyretin amyloidosis? What should be done next?

Pause and think before you click the answer:

Answer: The patient is suspected of having amyloid. A negative M band does not exclude amyloidosis. The patient's tongue is shown below. Though this is not highly typical, macroglossia is usually seen in AL amyloidosis only. There are clinical pointers to AL amyloidosis in this case such as macroglossia, rapid progression of the disease, and hypogammaglobulinemia. Eventually, a trephine biopsy showed myeloma and free light chain were markedly elevated (free lambda light chain 2,220 mg/L, free kappa chain 12.6 mg/L, total kappa lambda chain ratio 1.5:1—clinching the diagnosing of a light chain myeloma). The patient had occult blood positive in stool and an endoscopic biopsy showed duodenal amyloid as well.

There is a suspicion of macroglossia because of the teeth marks on the margins **(Fig. 4A)**, but a more typical picture is shown below from other patients with myeloma and amyloidosis **(Fig. 4B)**.

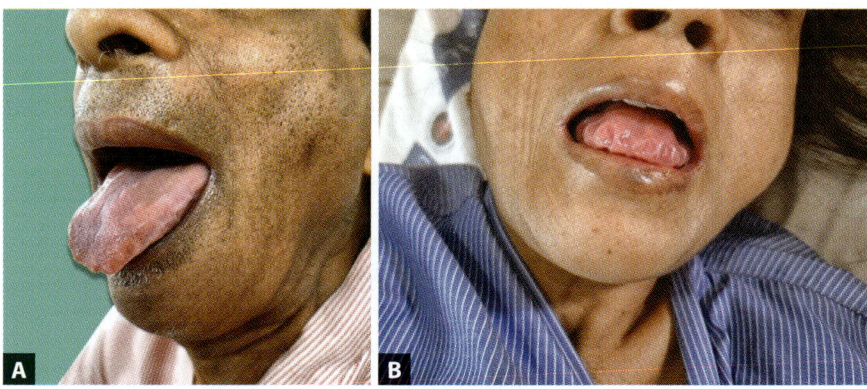

Figs. 4A and B: (A) The index patient; (B) Another patient with AL amyloidosis showing more typical macroglossia with dental impressions on the tongue (other details not shown).

- A third patient, a 38-year-old diabetic, hypothyroid lady started having breathlessness, atypical chest pain, and facial puffiness for the last 2–3 months. Subsequently, she developed acute renal failure with a creatinine of 10 mg/dL and required a few hemodialyses, and the renal failure recovered, but the symptoms of breathlessness persisted. Her chest X-ray and ECG are shown in **Figures 5 and 6**.

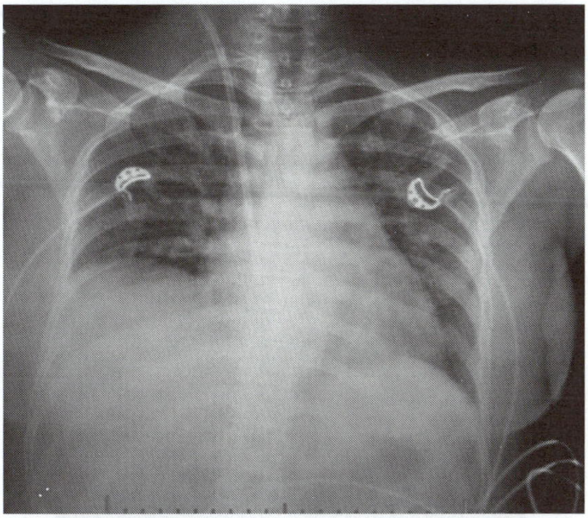

Fig. 5: Chest X-ray.

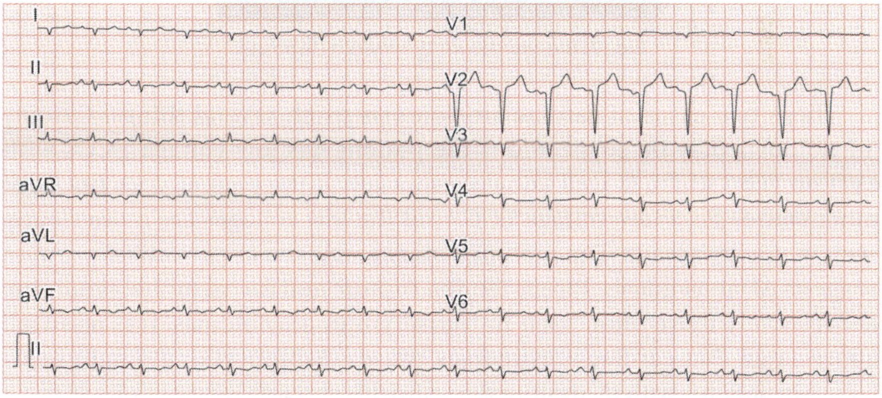

Fig. 6: ECG of the patient—low voltages in limb leads and poor progression of R waves.

Evaluation by echocardiography suggested the possibility of amyloidosis like the previous patient [left ventricular hypertrophy (LVH) on echo, low voltages on ECG, an episode of acute renal failure]. She had 5% plasma cells on bone marrow examination. M band was not seen. A cardiac biopsy **(Fig. 7)** showed an amyloid deposit and immunostaining confirmed AL amyloid. Subsequently, after 2 months, repeat bone marrow showed 11% plasma cells and she was being treated for myeloma.

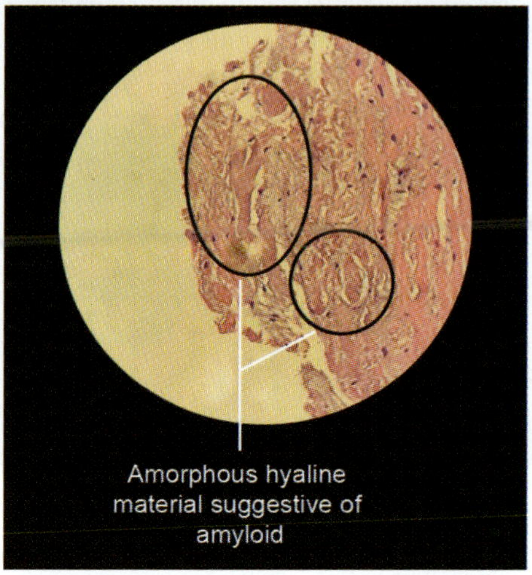

Fig. 7: Biopsy showing amyloid deposits.

These two cases of cardiac amyloidosis teach several things. Cardiac amyloidosis may be suspected if the patient has low-voltage ECGs with LVH on echo which is well known, especially if the patient does not have other causes for a low-voltage ECG, and the low voltages are more clearly seen in the limb leads. The presence of macroglossia or periorbital purpura suggests AL amyloidosis. Biceps tendon rupture and carpal tunnel syndrome are relatively more often seen in transthyretin amyloidosis. It is less well appreciated that cardiac amyloidosis causes disproportionate right heart failure in patients with LV dysfunction, and this should also make one suspect amyloidosis. (Both these patients had a tricuspid regurgitation that was not expected from the pulmonary artery pressures and such a right heart failure is commonly seen in cardiac amyloidosis that is disproportionate to left heart failure.) (**Video 3** from the first patient).

Video 3

Further, the fact that AL amyloidosis may happen without an M band, and without a myeloma diagnosis should also be kept in mind. (Amyloidosis and myeloma share a common causal root, namely, the presence of clonal malignant plasma cells in the bone marrow, but the behavior of these cells differs, leading to different clinical consequences. In amyloidosis, clonal plasma cells do not accumulate but induce the deposition of light chains in various organs as amyloid fibrils. The deposition of amyloid fibrils is independent of the tumor burden, whereas, in the myeloma, clonal plasma cells accumulate in the bone marrow, leading to anemia and bone destruction, among other harmful effects: Only 15% of myeloma patients have amyloidosis). We need evidence of monoclonal protein in the serum or urine, thus serum immunofixation, urine immunofixation, and free light chains ratio should be obtained in all patients. An excess of either free kappa or free lambda compared to the other indicates monoclonal proliferation. (Renal failure may alter the ratio even without amyloidosis!). A Tc PyP scan is usually positive in only transthyretin amyloid. Immunocharacterization of the type of amyloid on the biopsy is possible but should be done by an experienced pathologist only, as false positives and false negatives occur.

Learning points: Cardiac amyloidosis should be diagnosed early. Macroglossia and periorbital bruising suggest AL amyloid. All AL amyloid is not multiple myeloma. Rarely, transthyretin amyloid may coexist with AL amyloid. Transthyretin amyloidosis is increasingly diagnosed in the elderly with aortic stenosis and heart failure, though not discussed here.

Sidelights:

1. **What is the most common cause of a low-voltage ECG?**
2. **What causes sudden death in amyloidosis?**
3. **Which cardiac drugs are to be carefully used in patients with cardiac amyloidosis and heart failure?**
4. **What are the causes of LGE in the subendocardium on MRI?**

(*Sidelights are food for thought—provided to increase your curiosity:* So as a rule, do not read these answers before you try to answer them yourself. The answers provided here are not intended to be exhaustive.)

Answer: The most common cause of low-voltage ECG would be coronary artery disease and previous myocardial infarction (MI). Of course, low voltages are seen in large pericardial effusion, obesity, lung disease, large pleural effusion, and sometimes without an apparent cause.

- Sudden death is not uncommon in amyloidosis. A less well-appreciated cause of sudden cardiac death (SCD) in amyloidosis is electromechanical dissociation—a pulseless electrical activity that cannot be treated by an implanted cardioverter defibrillator. Of course, ventricular arrhythmias, conduction system disease, severe autonomic dysfunction, and pulmonary or systemic thromboembolism could also cause SCD.
- Patients with amyloidosis are sensitive to digoxin, and calcium channel blockers as these agents bind to amyloidosis. These patients also do not tolerate angiotensin-converting enzyme inhibitors (ACEi), angiotensin receptor blockers (ARB), and β-blockers.
- MRI showing subendocardial LGE typical of amyloidosis (**Fig. 8**, arrow). Such subendocardial LGE is also seen in patients with subendocardial ischemia, progressive systemic sclerosis, postcardiac transplantation, and rarely in myocarditis.

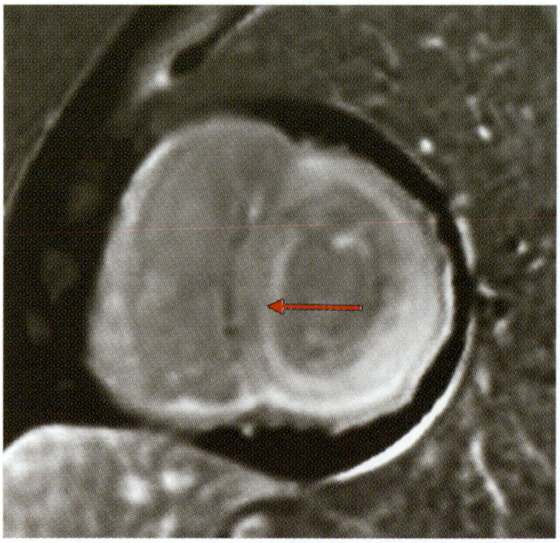

Fig. 8: Diffuse, near circumferential, and late gadolinium enhancement (arrow).

CASE

29

Mitral Stenosis

"Two things fill the mind with ever-increasing wonder and awe, the more often and the more intensely the mind of thought is drawn to them: the starry heavens above me and the moral law within me."

—Immanuel Kant

A 54-year-old male patient presented with recent onset progressive dyspnea on exertion (NYHA Class III) of 2 months duration associated with dry cough. There was no history of angina, syncope, prolonged fever, or previous heart disease. The patient was diagnosed with severe mitral stenosis with a dilated left atrium and large LA clot at a peripheral center and referred for further management.

His X-ray and ECG are shown in **Figures 1 and 2**.

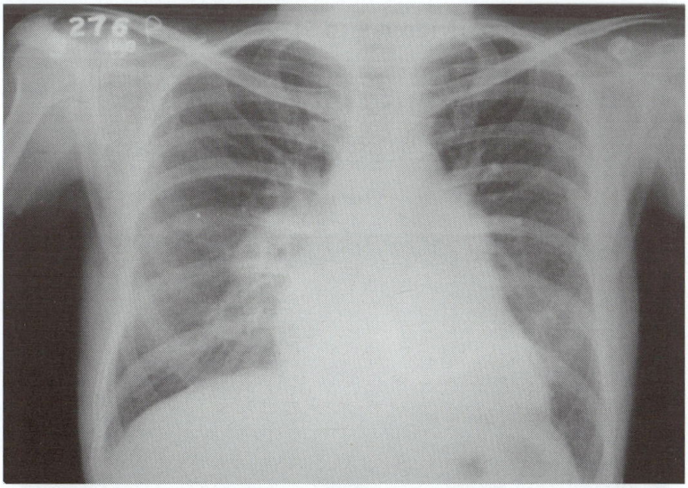

Fig. 1: Chest X-ray.

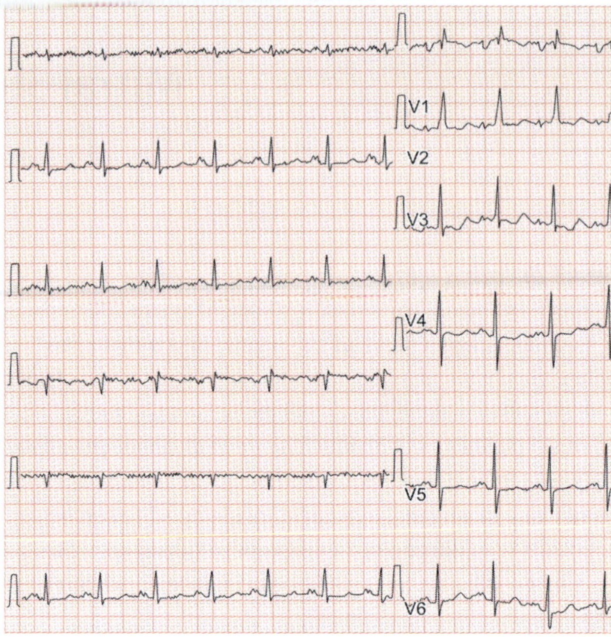

Fig. 2: ECG.

The echo is shown here **(Videos 1 to 3)**.

Video 1 Video 2 Video 3

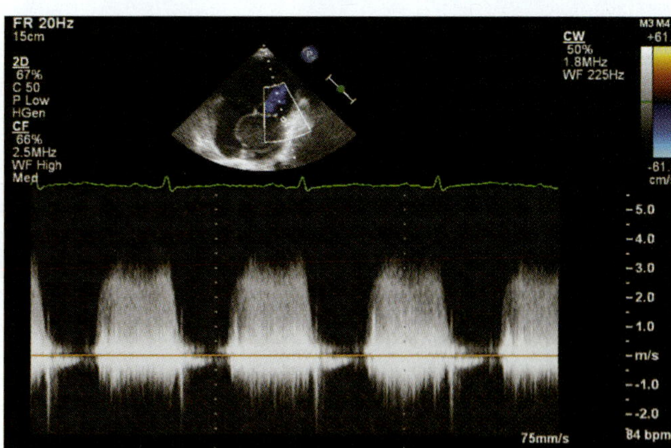

Fig. 3: Doppler across mitral valve showing left ventricular (LV) inflow obstruction.

There does not seem to be any doubt about mitral valve obstruction **(Fig. 3)**. See the detailed echo.

What is the likely possibility after viewing the echo?

Pause and think before you click the answer:

Answer: The transesophageal echocardiogram (TEE) shows the diagnosis **(Videos 4 and 5)**.

Video 4 **Video 5**

The patient has a left ventricular (LV) inflow obstruction from a large aneurysm of the sinus of Valsalva from the noncoronary sinus projecting into the left atrium. The patient was successfully operated. The aneurysm was resected and patched. The mitral valve was normal. It is important to think laterally when faced with an unusual situation. (obvious is obvious, look somewhere else.)

(*Source:* Selvaraj T, Malik V, Kiran U, Palaniswamy C. Unusual cause of acute pulmonary edema: unruptured aneurysm of noncoronary sinus causing severe mitral obstruction. Circ Heart Fail. 2009;2(4):382-5.)

See another mitral stenosis briefly.

- This 14-year-old girl presented with exertional breathlessness 3 years after a heart operation. The patient was operated for severe mitral regurgitation previously. All features now suggested severe mitral stenosis.

  The echo is shown here **(Video 6)**.

Video 6

What is the reason for mitral stenosis?

Again, pause and think before you click the answer:

Answer: It is an old echo record but shows the issue at hand well. The patient had undergone a mitral valve repair using a Duran ring for myxomatous mitral valve. The patient had an inflammatory response to the ring with a pannus formation that caused inflow obstruction; the mitral valve was normal. She was operated with ring resection only. The pannus is shown in **Figure 4**.

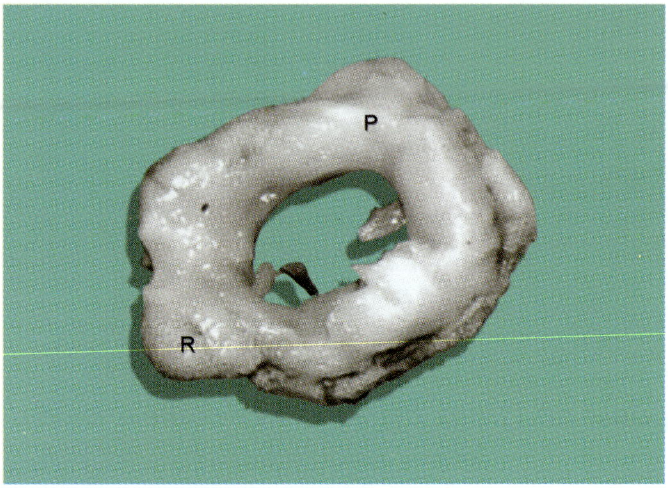

Fig. 4: Pannus around the mitral ring removed at operation.
(*Source:* Bisoi AK, Rajesh MR, Talwar S, Chauhan S, Ray R, Venugopal P. Mitral stenosis after Duran ring annuloplasty for non-rheumatic mitral regurgitation—a foreign body response? Heart Lung Circ. 2006;15(3):189-90.)

And yet another:

- A patient was referred for balloon mitral valvuloplasty. The echo is shown below **(Video 7)**.

Video 7

Answer: Rather nice demonstration of a supramitral ring for those who have not yet seen one. It is good to identify the supramitral ring as these patients might be operated easily. Beware of the association of a ring and congenital valve abnormalities as well.

- And further bonus—a rare variant of mitral stenosis—mitral arcade in a child **(Videos 8 and 9)**.

Video 8 Video 9

Anomalous mitral valve arcade is characterized by the connection of the LV papillary muscles to the anterior mitral leaflet, either directly or through the interposition of unusually short, thick, poorly differentiated chordae. Narrow spaces may be present between the abnormal chordae. It would not be treatable by balloon dilatation and is also a difficult lesion to repair surgically. Hence, it is important to recognize the abnormal anatomy.

(*Source:* Deepti S, Devagourou V, Kothari SS. Repair of anomalous mitral arcade in a child. Ann Pediatr Cardiol. 2017;10(2):200-2.)

Learning points: Left ventricular inflow obstruction may occur from a variety of pathologies. Even seemingly typical mitral stenosis needs to be viewed carefully.

Sidelights:

1. **Can there be a double orifice mitral valve from rheumatic heart disease (RHD)?**
2. **Can there be two mitral valves in a heart?**

(*Sidelights are food for thought—provided to increase your curiosity:* So as a rule, do not read these answers before you try to answer them yourself. The answers provided here are not intended to be exhaustive.)

Answer: Double orifice mitral valve due to uneven commissural fusion can occur in RHD, and balloon dilatation of such mitral valve using two smaller-sized Inoue balloons has been reported. Alternatively, a patient with a congenitally double orifice mitral valve might develop RHD and commissural fusion.

- Two mitral valves in a heart leading to a total of three AV valves have been described. Such hearts commonly have double outlet left atrium.

CASE

30

Some Fevers

"Every truth has two sides; it is as well to look at both, before we commit ourselves to either."

—Aesop

A 10-year-old child had a fever for 2 weeks and the following X-ray **(Fig. 1)**. He has effort limitation since early childhood but has not been evaluated. Can you guess the diagnosis? If not obvious, only then see the hint.

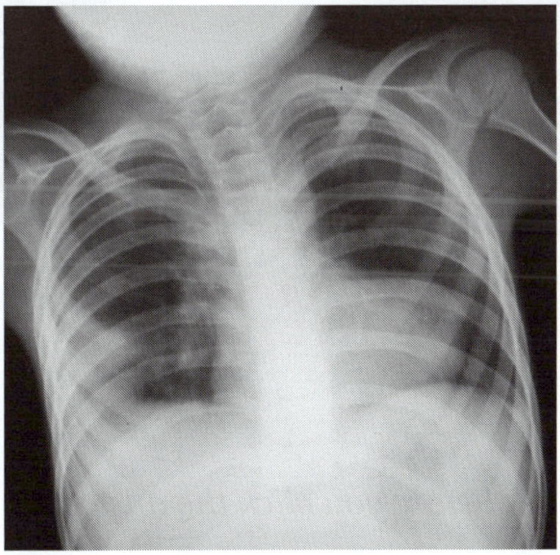

Fig. 1: Chest X-ray.

(Hint: The child has a cyanotic congenital heart disease.)

If you could not diagnose, then see this X-ray of another child with fever due to recurrent pneumonia from a similar illness (Fig. 2). What are the similarities and differences between the two children's diseases?

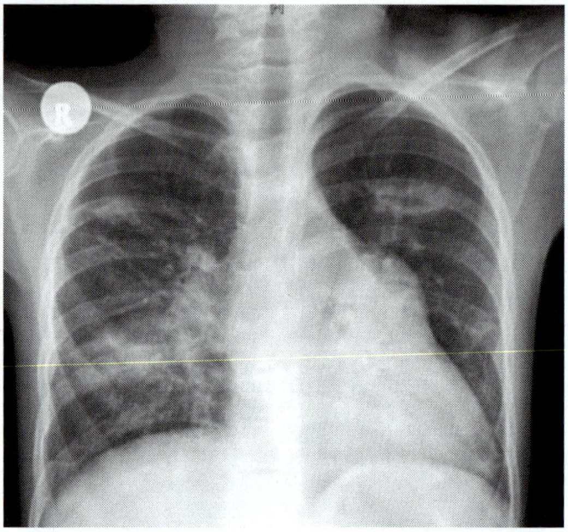

Fig. 2: Chest X-ray of another child.

Pause and think before you click the answer:

Answer: Both have right-sided infective endocarditis (IE) and congenital heart disease. The first child has a typical tetralogy of Fallot (TOF) X-ray and a pulmonary infarct. In the setting of fever, a right-sided IE should be considered. The second child had a ventricular septal defect (VSD), increased pulmonary blood flow, and endocarditis on the right side where the VSD jet strikes the RV wall. The chest X-ray again shows infiltrates in the lungs from septic emboli. It is not uncommon to see such patients being treated only as recurrent pneumonia and missing IE, hence the presentation here.

- Now look at this 20-year-old young adult with similar congenital heart disease having fever for 1 month duration. What is the diagnosis **(Fig. 3)**?

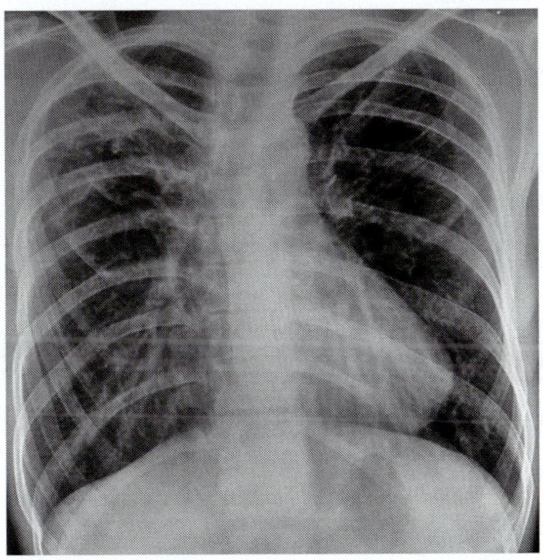

Fig. 3: Chest X-ray of an adult with congenital heart disease (CHD) and fever.

Answer: Tuberculosis is more common in patients with TOF possibly. The reasons are not very clear, but it is hypothesized that *Mycobacteria*, an aerobic bacteria, may thrive better in lung apices with pulmonary oligemia. It has not been well researched if this is true, but the clinical experience does seem to favor the fact that tuberculosis in CHD (more so in CHD with reduced pulmonary blood flow like TOF) is more common than in the general population. In any case, the chest X-ray shows tuberculosis in the apex (something the cardiology residents often miss to look at).

Learning points: Recurrent pneumonia in a child with heart disease could result from right-sided IE.

Tuberculosis may occur more commonly in a cyanotic child with decreased pulmonary blood flow.

Sidelights: What are the mimics of vegetations?

(*Sidelights are food for thought—provided to increase your curiosity:* So as a rule, do not read these answers before you try to answer them yourself. The answers provided here are not intended to be exhaustive.)

Answer: It cannot be overemphasized that IE remains a clinical diagnosis. Echo is extremely useful in the diagnosis of IE, yet there are numerous mimics and masquerades of vegetations. Libman-Sacks endocarditis (noninfectious vegetation), fibroelastoma, Chiari malformation, thrombus, accessory valve tissue, tumor masses, sutures, ruptured chordae, artefacts, prolapsed leaflets, Lambl's excrescence, and many other lesions may appear like a vegetation. Uncommonly, hypereosinophilic syndrome **(Figs. 4A and B)**, Wegener's granulomatosis, and Behçet's disease may produce masses simulating vegetation.

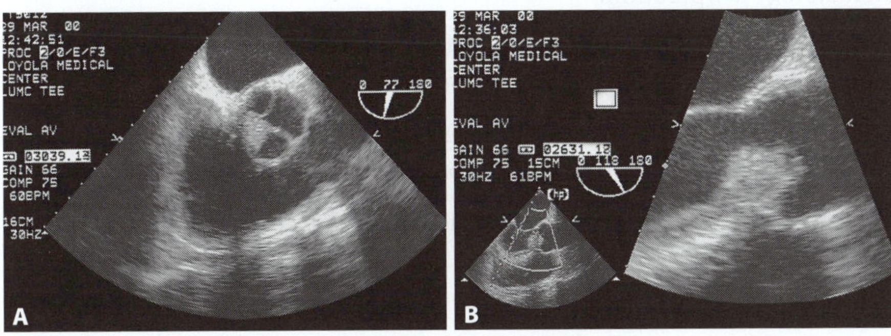

Figs. 4A and B: Hypereosinophilic syndrome (from open source, exact source—not known).

Which of the following videos shows vegetations? Try to diagnose the abnormality shown in the video before seeing the answers.

Video 1 Video 2 Video 3 Video 4

Video 5 Video 6 Video 7 Video 8

Answer:

Video 1: A metastatic PNET tumor appearing like vegetation. (Clinical details are needed for the diagnosis.)

Video 2: Accessory tricuspid valve tissue in a patient of TOF, no vegetation.

Video 3: Another accessory tissue, no vegetation (old record).

Video 4: Acute rheumatic fever with chordal rupture, no vegetation.

Video 5: Patient of severe AR with a nodule on the aortic valve. No vegetation on histology at operation.

Video 6: These are ghosts after a pacemaker lead has been removed. Do not indicate infection. (From web open source).

Video 7: Libman sacks endocarditis [systemic lupus erythematosus (SLE) and antiphospholipid antibodies (APLA) positive], no IE.

Video 8: Neonate with spontaneous tricuspid valve chordal rupture, no IE.

CASE

31

Cardiac Masses

"To ask the "right" question is far more important than to receive the answer. The solution of a problem lies in the understanding of the problem; the answer is not outside the problem, it is in the problem."

—J Krishnamurthy

A 3-year-old child had abdominal distention for the past 4 months. He developed facial puffiness also for the last 1 month and was referred for an echo. He had no illness previously. His echo is shown here **(Videos 1 to 3)**.

Video 1

Video 2

Video 3

What is the diagnosis?

Pause and think before you click the answer:

Answer: The first echo is suspicious of an RA mass, possibly a myxoma that is prolapsing through the tricuspid valve in the second echo. However, the third video clearly shows that the mass is an extension from the inferior vena cava (IVC). Wilm's tumor is known to have extension en mass to the heart. A preoperative chemotherapy generally leads to a reduction of the IVC mass and facilitates surgical resection of the tumor en bloc. Cure can be obtained in patients with IVC extension in Wilm's tumor with modern-day chemotherapy.

The approach to intracardiac masses in echo is interesting. Tissue characterization by magnetic resonance imaging (MRI) is often required in uncertain situations. But, the interpretation is often facilitated by the clinical context.

Rather old poor echo record that represents an interesting disease.

- This echo is from a 12-year-old malnourished child with a fever of 3 months duration **(Video 4)**.

Video 4

What is the likely diagnosis?

Pause and think before you click the answer:

Answer: This RA mass in a febrile malnourished child was a tuberculoma. The patient had military tuberculosis so the diagnosis was not difficult. In other similar patients, sometimes a biopsy of the mass may be required, if there is doubt after a clinical evaluation and MRI.

- A 12-year-old boy had progressive exertional fatigue and palpitations for the last 1 year. He had no fever, weight loss, or history of chest trauma. He had a normal cardiovascular examination except for mildly elevated jugular venous pressure (JVP). The chest X-ray showed mild cardiomegaly, but the ECG was abnormal **(Fig. 1)**. It showed RBBB with saddle-shaped ST elevation like a Brugada syndrome. The echo showed an infiltrating mass surrounding both the right and left ventricles, mostly around the outflow tracts. The infiltrating mass was better characterized on MRI. (See legends of **Figures 2A to E** for details).

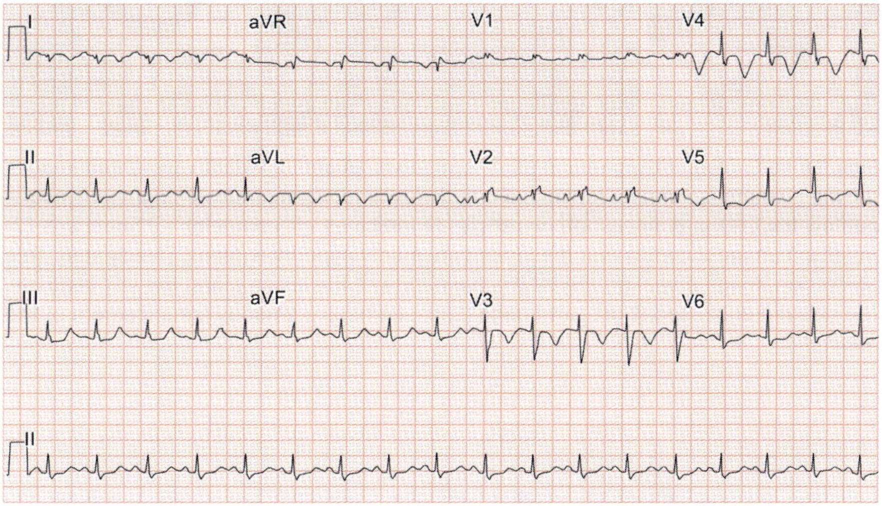

Fig. 1: ECG showing incomplete right bundle branch block (RBBB) and diffuse ST-T changes. (Note the saddle-shaped elevation in V1 like in Brugada syndrome).

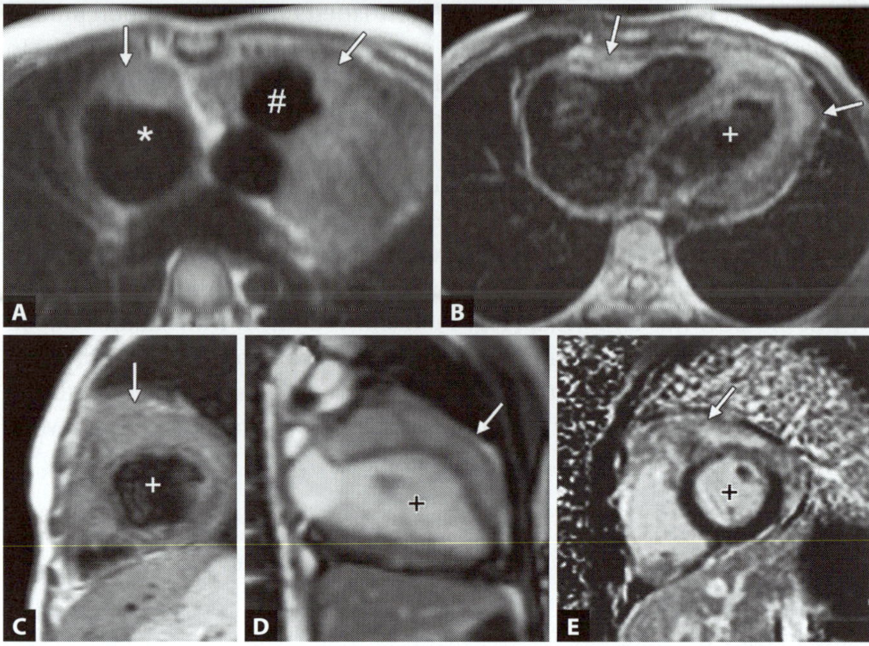

Figs. 2A to E: Cardiac magnetic resonance images. (A and B) Axial T1-weighted images showing isointense masses (arrows) along the anterior right atrium (*), right ventricular outflow tract (#), and along both ventricles (+ indicates left ventricle); (C) Short axis T2-weighted image showing that the lesions are mildly hyperintense; (D) Steady state-free precession image revealing the infiltrative nature of the lesion along the left ventricle. The delayed enhanced short-axis image (E) shows heterogeneous enhancement of the mass.

Why does the ECG show epsilon waves? What is the likely diagnosis?

Pause and think before you click the answer:

Answer: The epicardial infiltration creates inhomogeneity in repolarization and gives epsilon waves. Such has been described in patients with lymphomatous infiltration of the heart also. The patient did not have mediastinal lymphadenopathy or fever, but we empirically gave him antitubercular therapy and the mass disappeared **(Fig. 3)**.

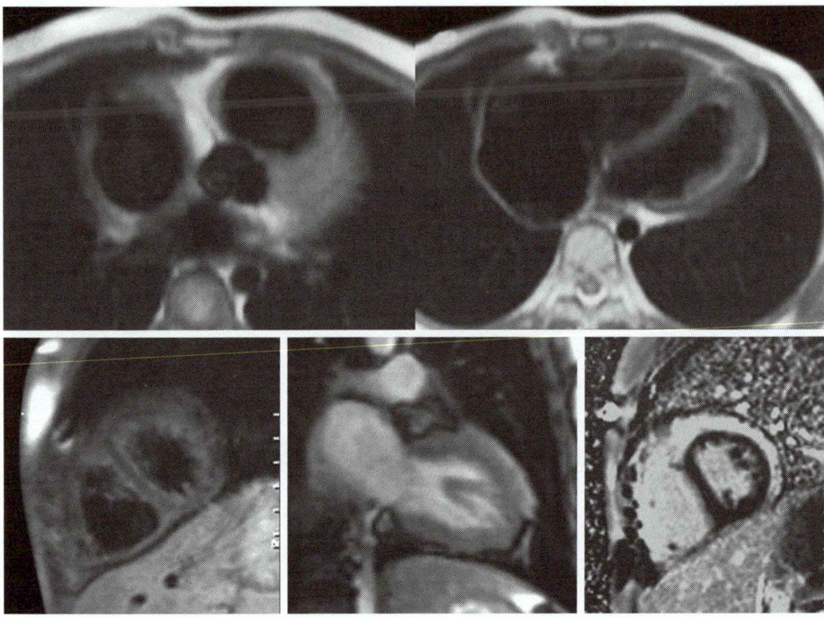

Fig. 3: Magnetic resonance imaging (MRI) after 6 months of antitubercular therapy shows significant reductions in all the lesions.

Bonus echo: A neonate with massive septal hypertrophy mimicking HCM, that turned out to be a hemangioma on MR imaging **(Videos 5 and 6)**.

Video 5 Video 6

- A 20-day-old neonate with heart failure and cyanosis with a massive cardiac tumor. He died before the planned debulking surgery could be done **(Videos 7 and 8)**. What is the diagnosis?

Video 7 Video 8

Obviously, this was a massive biventricular rhabdomyoma. Rhabdomyoma regress spontaneously and also with mTOR inhibitors such as everolimus.

Learning points: The approach to cardiac masses is interesting. There are some spot diagnoses based on the echo picture. More often, it is the total context, as always, that will decide. Of course, tissue characterization by MRI is very useful.

Sidelights: How to distinguish thrombus from myxoma?

(*Sidelights are food for thought—provided to increase your curiosity:* So as a rule, do not read these answers before you try to answer them yourself. The answers provided here are not intended to be exhaustive.)

Answer: Generally clinical context would be able to distinguish the two. Occasionally, the distinction may be difficult. Lack of vascularity with delayed inversion time and no LGE on MRI favors a thrombus. But it should be remembered that 2% of tumors might not be vascular, and sometimes a large tumor gets necrosis in the center and may be avascular. Or the thrombus might get neovascularized and show enhancement. A myxoma might have a thrombus attached to it or may get infected and have vegetations within it.

Case 31A: Mitral Regurgitation and a Mass

A 24-year-old man had dyspnea and palpitations for the last 2 months that had rapidly progressed to class 4. There was no history of fever, joint pains, skin rash, or weight loss. On examination, he was in heart failure and had a mitral regurgitation murmur. His routine biochemistry tests were normal. His echo showed severe mitral regurgitation (MR) and a mass in the left ventricle.

See the accompanying videos **(Videos 9 and 10)** and the pictures in **Figures 4 and 5**.

Video 9 Video 10

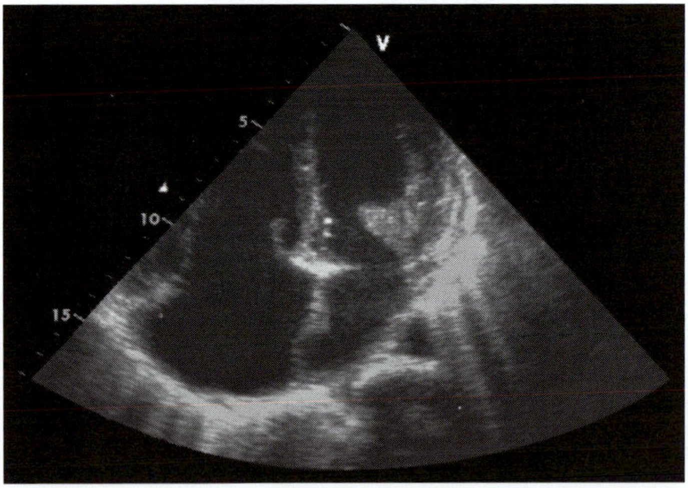

Fig. 4: The mass in the left ventricle.

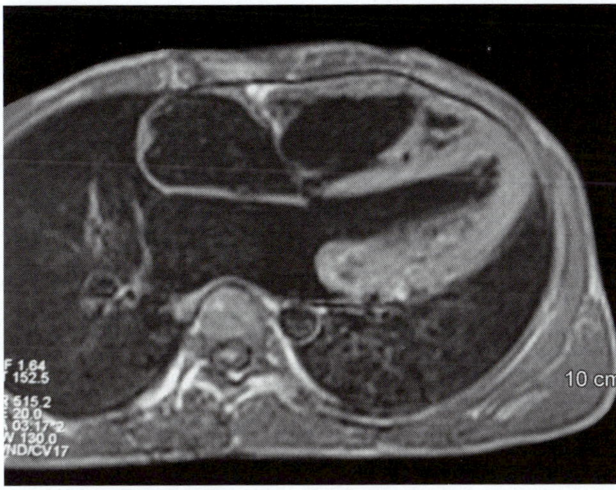

Fig. 5: Contrast-enhanced MRI showing a posteromedial mass involving the mitral valve apparatus.

The MRI showed the mass was isointense relative to the myocardium on the T1-weighted images and minimally hyperintense on the T2-weighted images. The mass showed homogenous enhancement after intravenous injection of gadolinium. On the basis of the MRI features, a benign mass, possibly of chronic inflammatory origin, was suspected.

What do you think should be done?

Pause and think before you click the answer:

Answer: Since the patient had severe MR and heart failure and a mass, he underwent surgery. The mass turned out to be an inflammatory mass from myocarditis. The resected tumor showed Aschoff`s nodules. The antistreptolysin O (ASLO) titer was 900 units. Acute rheumatic fever is not expected to cause much myocardial involvement. In fact, there is no significant myocardial involvement in acute rheumatic fever, and there is primarily mostly only valvulitis in rheumatic fever. Valve replacement in patients with severe heart failure in acute rheumatic fever has resulted in prompt clinical improvement in some reports because there is no myocardial issue.

This patient did not have any clinical features suggesting rheumatic fever. However, the Aschoff's nodules are typically seen only in rheumatic fever. Hence, the final impression was that rarely, rheumatic fever might cause myocardial involvement as seen in this patient. Whether the patient could have responded to steroids and a mitral valve replacement could have been avoided remains unknown.

Remember pseudotumor when faced with a tumor.

The resected mitral valve and the surrounding myocardial mass showed Aschoff's nodule **(Figs. 6 and 7)**.

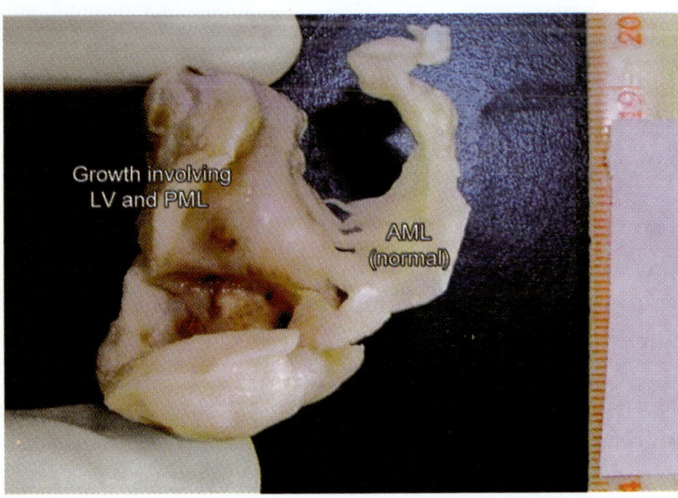

Fig. 6: Resected specimen.

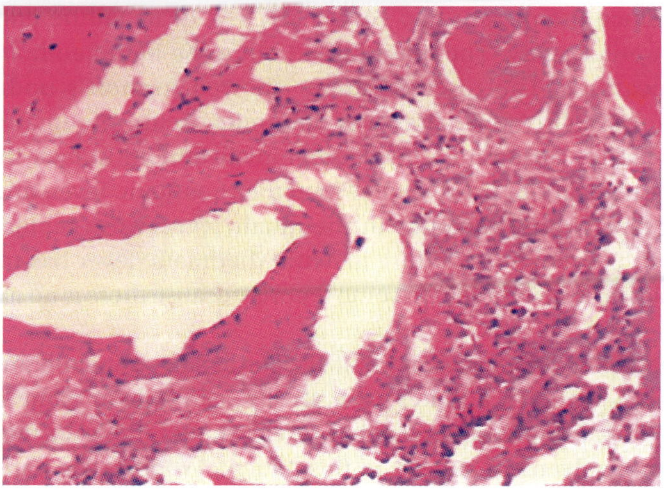

Fig. 7: The histology of the resected mass showed Aschoff's nodule.

(*Source:* Kothari SS, Bisoi AK, Singh S, Gulati G, Varshnay S, Ray R. Rheumatic myocarditis masquerading as left ventricle tumor. Circulation. 2006;114(11):e487-8.)

Learning points: Generally, rheumatic fever does not have significant myocardial involvement and heart failure is the result of valvular involvement.

Sidelights:

1. **What is the echo evidence of active rheumatic fever?**
2. **How to diagnose chronic rheumatic carditis?**

(*Sidelights are food for thought—provided to increase your curiosity:* So as a rule, do not read these answers before you try to answer them yourself. The answers provided here are not intended to be exhaustive.)

Answer: Active rheumatic fever is a clinical diagnosis. The cardiac involvement in the ARF may lead to new onset regurgitation and pericardial effusion. Lesser known facets of rheumatic fever include mitral valve prolapse (due to chordal inflammation, annulitis, and leaflet involvement), the presence of tiny rheumatic nodules on the mitral and aortic valve with regurgitation, and annular dysfunction. Chordal rupture rarely may occur in ARF. In the case of chronic rheumatic heart disease (RHD), a change in the picture denoting any of the above may indicate active rheumatic fever.

- Chronic rheumatic carditis is a clinical diagnosis empirically employed in children with a prolonged course of rheumatic fever. There are no clear diagnostic criteria but the clinical impression of continuing activity by the constitutional features and raised inflammatory markers often in a child with congestive heart failure and significant mitral/aortic regurgitation.

The video below show the rheumatic nodules in patients with acute rheumatic fever **(Videos 11 and 12)**.

Video 11 Video 12

CASE

32

Cyanosis at 69 Years

"Knowing is not enough; we must apply.
Willing is not enough; we must do."

—Johann Wolfgang von Goethe

A 69-year-old lady developed breathlessness on exertion for the last 6 months and had pedal edema and cyanosis of recent origin for the last 4 months. She had a history of intermittent loose stools for 3 months and an abdominal ovarian mass for 3 months. The saturation in room air was 79%. She was in heart failure with severe tricuspid regurgitation (TR). The ECG and X-ray are shown in **Figures 1 and 2**. The patient complained of worsening of symptoms on getting up and the saturation was 2–3% worse on getting up.

Why would anyone develop central cyanosis at 69 years of age?

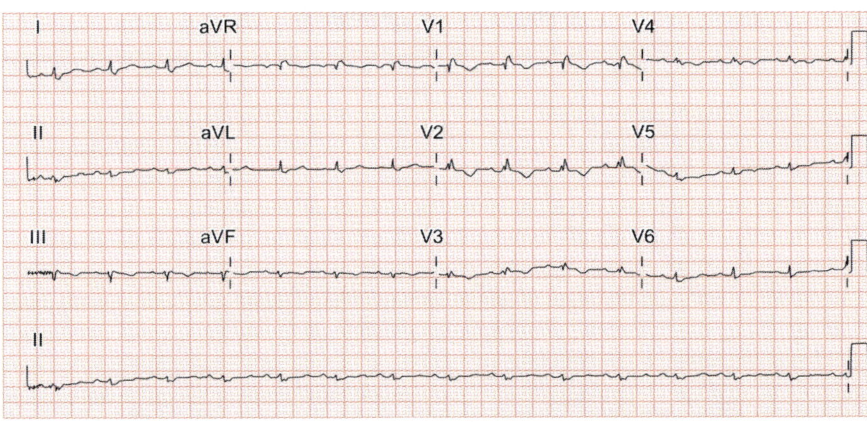

Fig. 1: ECG showing complete right bundle branch block (RBBB).

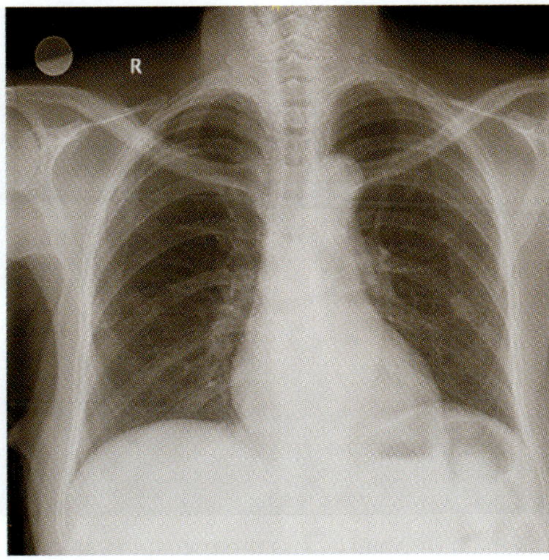

Fig. 2: Chest X-ray.

The echo videos are shown here **(Videos 1 to 5)**.

Video 1 **Video 2** **Video 3**

Video 4 **Video 5**

She was noticed to have significant TR, mild tricuspid stenosis **(Fig. 3)**, mitral regurgitation, and moderate aortic regurgitation. The interatrial septum appeared intact, but careful examination and a contrast echo showed a right to left shunt through a small atrial septal defect (ASD)/patent foramen ovale (PFO) (Video 5).

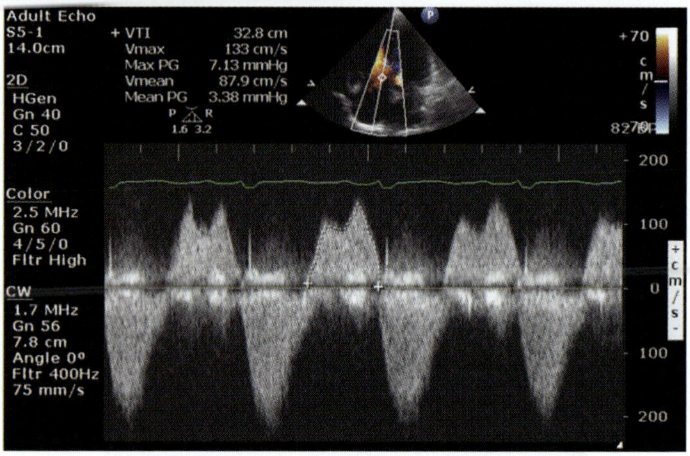

Fig. 3: Doppler across the tricuspid valve.

The abdominal mass was an ovarian mass. The liver was normal.

What is the diagnosis? What tests are required?

Pause and think before you click the answer:

Answer: Acquired central cyanosis at the age of 67 suggests an acquired TR and a right to left shunt through an ASD. The plate-like tricuspid valve morphology is highly suspicious of a carcinoid syndrome (Video 1). When there is an ASD with carcinoid syndrome, it may cause left-sided valvar lesions such as MR and AR as in this case (Video 3). The change in tricuspid jet with posture possibly accounted for the platypnea-orthodeoxia symptoms in her case. The 67 Dotanac and the MRI **(Figs. 4 and 5)** showed an ovarian mass but no metastasis. The urinary 5-HIAA levels were normal. The histology of the resected tumor showed a neuroendocrine tumor, consistent with the diagnosis of carcinoid syndrome. A tricuspid bioprosthesis was placed, and the ovarian carcinoid cyst was removed. The histology of the resected ovarian tumor was consistent with carcinoid syndrome. In contrast to Gut carcinoid, ovarian carcinoid can cause carcinoid syndrome without liver metastasis as the ovarian blood drains directly to the inferior vena cava!

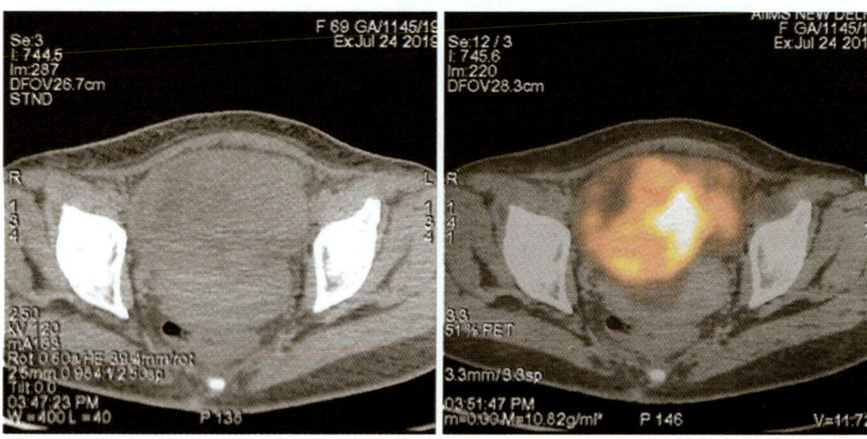

Fig. 4: ^{68}GA Dotanac whole-body PET-CT showing ovarian mass.

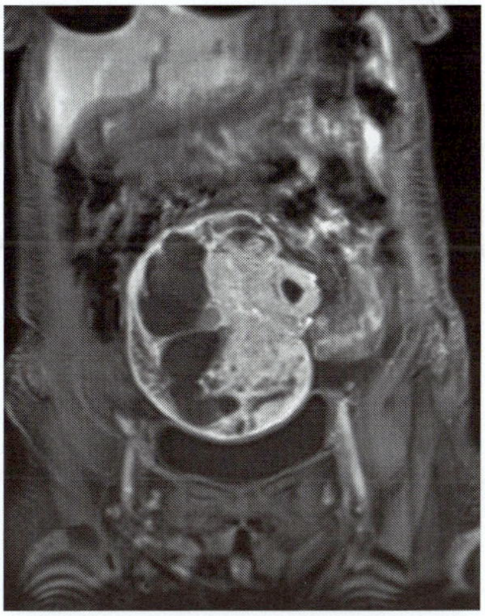

Fig. 5: Magnetic resonance imaging (MRI) abdomen and pelvis—the mass is showing arterial hyperenhancement with progressive filling in of contrast in the venous and delayed phases. The central part of the mass is showing areas of necrosis.

Learning points: The typical tricuspid valve plate-like morphology is the clue to the diagnosis of Carcinoid syndrome.

Carcinoid syndrome in the presence of an ASD (or with lung metastasis/bronchial carcinoid) may cause left-sided valve lesions confusing the picture.

Rarely, ovarian tumors can cause carcinoid syndrome.

Sidelights: What diseases may cause flushing?

(*Sidelights are food for thought—provided to increase your curiosity:* So as a rule, do not read these answers before you try to answer them yourself. The answers provided here are not intended to be exhaustive.)

Answer: Flushing increased warmth and reddening of skin may be episodic or persistent. The disorders to keep in mind beyond the simple (menopause, emotions or fever, alcohol, drugs, or food, and rosacea) are carcinoid syndrome, anaphylaxis, pheochromocytoma, mastocytosis, neuroendocrine tumors, medullary thyroid cancer, Cushing syndrome, renal cell carcinoma, Fabry disease, autonomic dysfunction, and rarely chronic aortic regurgitation.

What is the cause of TR in this patient (Fig. 6)?

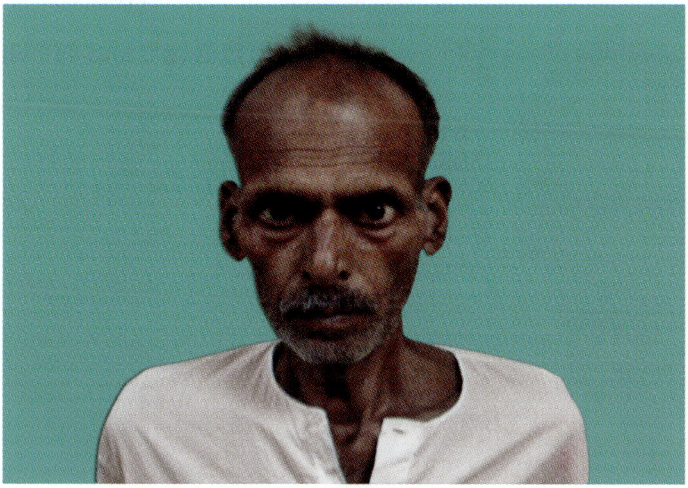

Fig. 6: Patient with TR (with permission).

Answer: Thyrotoxicosis is a less well-recognized cause of TR!

Bonus video:
See the video of a 69-day-old infant with TR **(Videos 6 and 7)**. What is the cause of TR?

Video 6 Video 7

Answer: The TR in neonates from chordal rupture. This was successfully repaired. No IE.

CASE

33

Congestive Heart Failure in Tetralogy of Fallot

"Truth is found neither in the thesis nor the antithesis, but in an emergent synthesis which reconciles the two."

—GWF Hegel

A 10-year-old child with tetralogy of Fallot (TOF) presented with severe cyanosis, exertional breathlessness, abdominal distention, and pedal edema. The child was previously diagnosed with TOF but had not undergone any treatment. On examination, heart rate 100 beats/min, blood pressure 110/80 mm Hg, cardiomegaly, and a short ejection systolic murmur of TOF were found. The child was in congestive heart failure (CHF) with raised jugular venous pressure (JVP), hepatomegaly, and ascites. His ECG was consistent with TOF. The chest X-ray is shown in **Figure 1**. The echo showed left ventricular ejection fraction (LVEF) of 22%. A cardiac catheterization showed the TOF anatomy with poor right and left ventricular function. The right atrial mean pressure was 18 mm Hg and the right ventricular and left ventricular end diastolic pressures were 17–20 mm Hg, respectively. There were no significant collaterals. There was no suggestion of viral myocarditis in the past or a family history of cardiomyopathy. The liver function test, renal function tests, and thyroid function tests were normal.

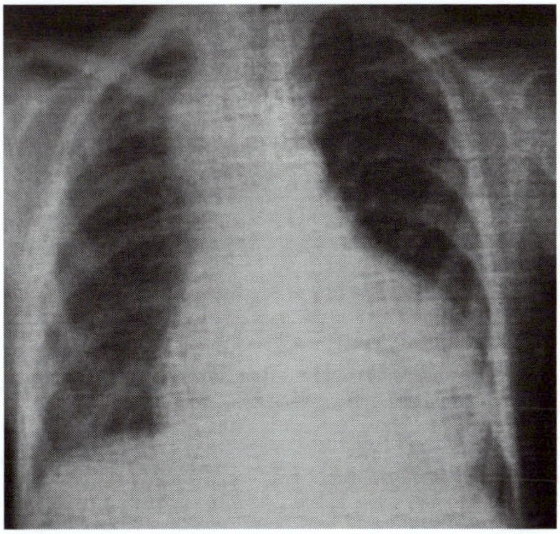

Fig. 1: Chest X-ray.

Why the patient is in heart failure? (His heart failure improved substantially after a procedure, and he underwent corrective surgery later.)

Pause and think before you click the answer:

Answer: Congestive heart failure typically does not occur in TOF as the volume ejected by combined ventricles is normal. If the demand on the heart is increased, or the cardiac contractility is diminished for some reasons, congestive cardiac failure might occur. The most common cause of heart failure in children with TOF is anemia. (It is important to realize that hemoglobin <14 g% is anemia for any cyanotic patient with saturation of 85% or less, and proportionately more hemoglobin is required with lesser saturations). Other causes include hypertension, valvular regurgitation (aortic or other valves), infective endocarditis, large volume loads following a Blalock-Taussig (BT) shunt, or aortopulmonary collaterals (which are very uncommon to cause heart failure, but students always remember these as a cause!), associated myocarditis, or cardiomyopathy, rheumatic heart disease, other causes of ventricular dysfunction as in any other setting like tachycardiomyopathy, hypocalcemia, myocardial ischemia from any cause, etc. Adult TOF patients often have reduced contractility from ventricular fibrosis due to ongoing insults of hypoxia, chronic pressure load, polycythemia, etc. TOF with absent pulmonary valve patients might be in heart failure from increased pulmonary blood flow, and TOF with restrictive ventricular septal defect has increased pressure load with suprasystemic right ventricle and might show heart failure. The hemoglobin in this patient was 22 g% and the saturation was only 54%. This information was not provided just to check whether you would think that hypoxia and polycythemia could be a cause of CHF. The patient improved markedly after a BT shunt of 6 mm that would have added additional volume load to the heart and would have caused heart failure instead! Only a few similar cases are described in the literature. The hypoxia has to be severe to cause ventricular dysfunction as the organs can autoregulate oxygen extraction to a large extent. Polycythemia is underrecognized as a cause of ventricular dysfunction, but it is difficult to separate its influence from that of hypoxia, and both might be responsible. The ventricualr function improved remarkably after the shunt, though it improved gradually over a few months! The LVEF 4 months after the shunt operation was 40%.

(*Source:* Chowdhury UK, Subramaniam GK, Kothari SS, Airan B, Venugopal P. Congestive heart failure in unoperated tetralogy of Fallot: can hypoxia be a cause? Indian Heart J. 2005;57(1):65-7.)

- *Another case of TOF and heart failure:* The chest X-ray **(Fig. 2)** and ECG **(Fig. 3)** of a 3-year-old patient with TOF and restrictive VSD are shown here. Can you identify the cause of CHF in him?

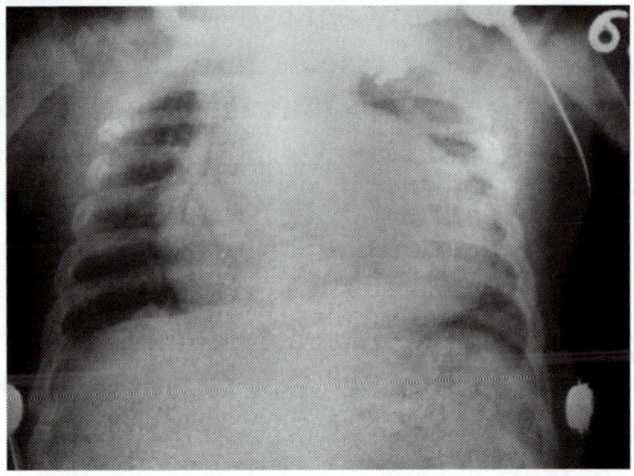

Fig. 2: Chest X-ray.

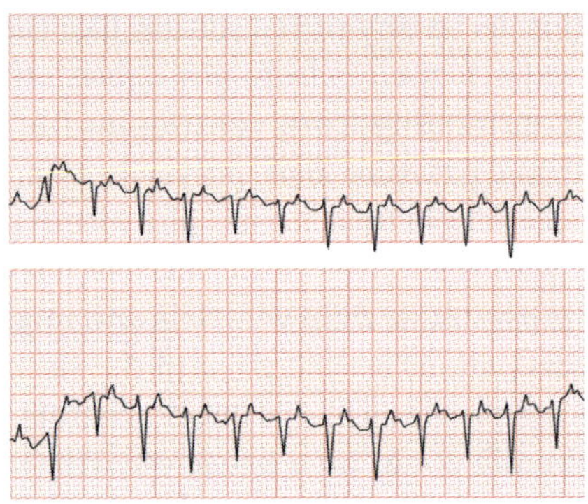

Fig. 3: ECG.

Pause and think before you click the answer:

Answer: The chest X-ray shows significant cardiomegaly. The patient has a restrictive VSD (as mentioned); such patients develop suprasystemic right ventricular pressure, tricuspid regurgitation, and heart failure. But what did the ECG show? Did you pick up the ectopic atrial tachycardia from the pointed P waves and prolonged PR interval for this heart rate? (The ECG is not at all typical of TOF, but such was the ECG in this case, perhaps related to placement issues or distortion from the dilated right atrium!). The heart failure is due to a combination of suprasystemic RV pressure and ectopic atrial tachycardia further causing ventricular dysfunction.

And another cause: What does **Video 1** show?

Video 1

Answer: The video is from a patient of TOF with hypertrophic cardiomyopathy (HCM). You can suspect that from the disproportionately thickened and echogenic interventricular septum. (Agreed that it is not clearly diagnostic in this instance, but the patient had HCM with TOF).

Learning points: Tetralogy of Fallot's patients rarely have CHF. Several causes of heart failure in TOF are taught. But, severe chronic hypoxia causing ventricular dysfunction is rarely appreciated. Hypoxia-induced ventricular dysfunction is uncommon and occurs only if the hypoxia is severe (possibly <60% saturation or below). Associated severe polycythemia might worsen the ventricular function more.

Sidelights:

1. **What is the effect of polycythemia on pulmonary vascular resistance?**
2. **Does blood transfusion in a child with anemia and TOF change the arterial saturation?**

(*Sidelights are food for thought—provided to increase your curiosity:* So as a rule, do not read these answers before you try to answer them yourself. The answers provided here are not intended to be exhaustive.)

Answer: The viscosity of blood doubles from a hematocrit of 40% (normal) to 60% (hemoglobin about 16 g%). Since the resistance to the flow in a tube depends on the length, radius, and the viscosity of fluid in it ($8\ \eta l/\pi r^4$), such a change might make an important difference in pulmonary vascular resistance, especially in low flow states such as in a Fontan circulation.

- Since anemia causes lowering of systemic vascular resistance, correction of anemia by increasing vascular resistance reduces the right to left shunt and thus increases pulmonary blood flow. Therefore, transfusion of packed cells to a child with TOF improves saturation significantly and ameliorates the symptoms markedly.

CASE

34

Exertional Syncope

"The young man knows the rules, but the old man knows the exceptions."
—Oliver Wendell Holmes, Sr.

A 52-year-old man presented with two episodes of syncope. He was a known hypertensive on irregular medication, a chronic tobacco chewer, and was accustomed to regular moderate alcohol consumption. Both the episodes were on exertion (first after straining at stool, the second while cycling) and were accompanied by sweating and palpitation before passing out. The patient spontaneously regained consciousness in both episodes within 2–3 minutes. The physical examination was unremarkable except for the nicotine stains on the teeth and mild hypertension with blood pressure of 145/90 mm Hg. The troponins were mildly elevated. (150 ng/mL, normal 14 ng/mL). The ECG showed borderline left ventricular hypertrophy (LVH) and <0.5 mm ST segment depression in lateral leads as shown in **Figure 1**.

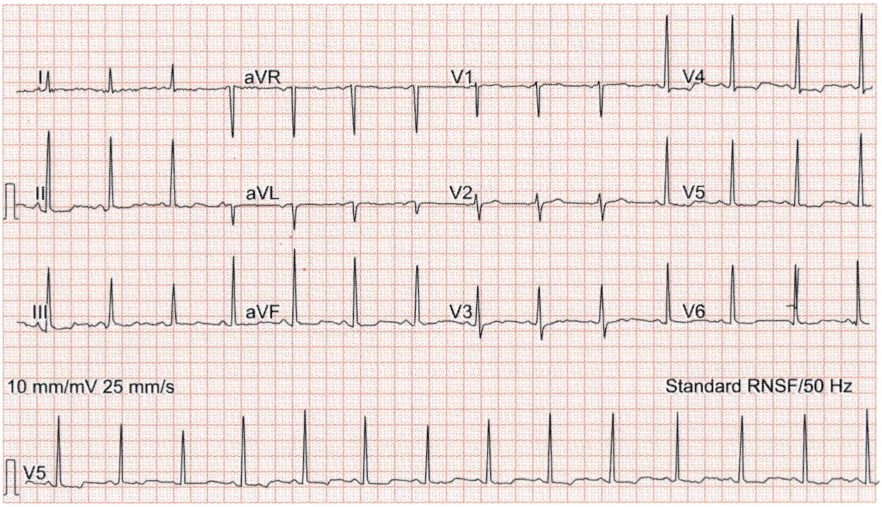

Fig. 1: ECG.

The echo videos are shown below **(Videos 1 and 2)**. The echo was interpreted as mild endocardial scarring, but no regional wall motion abnormality.

Video 1 Video 2

A coronary angio was done **(Video 3)**.

Video 3

A cardiac magnetic resonance imaging (MRI) was ordered as the MRI facility was recently acquired and that showed no features of cardiac sarcoidosis, normal LV function, and stress MRI done with adenosine was normal. There was no late gadolinium enhancement (LGE).

What should be done next?

Pause and think before you click the answer:

Answer: This case illustrates the value of selecting the right test for investigation. The background and clinical history are very suggestive of coronary artery disease (CAD). A coronary angiogram was not properly interpreted and the CAD was thought not to account for the symptoms. Fractional flow reserve (FFR) was not possible due to logistics reasons. The angiogram might miss a lesion or lesion severity due to a number of reasons. The patient had a treadmill test (TMT) done before discharge. The TMT is shown below. At 5 METs of exercise, the patient had angina and the ST elevation **(Fig. 2)**.

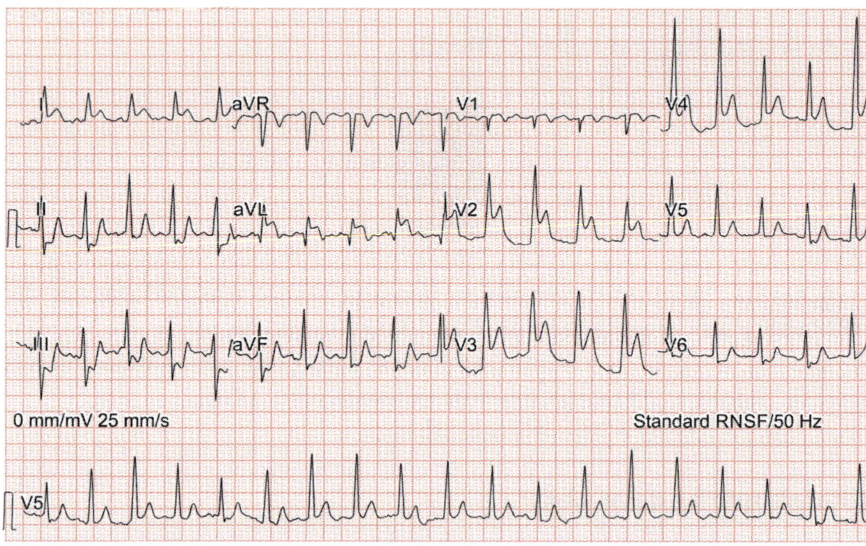

Fig. 2: ECG during a treadmill test at low workload.

A repeat coronary angiogram showed a tight LAD lesion (**Video 4** and **Fig. 3**).

Video 4

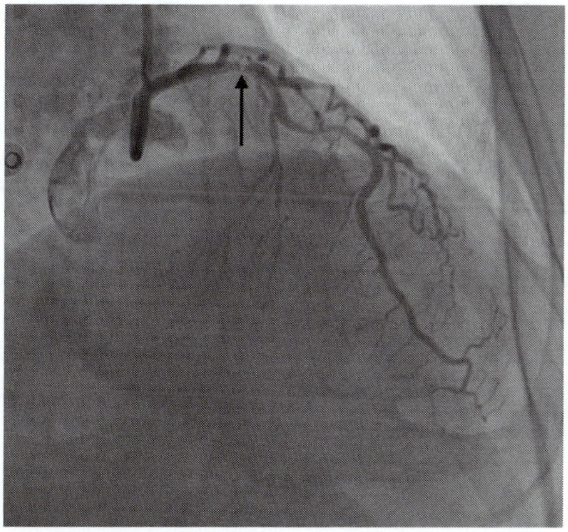

Fig. 3: Repeat coronary angiogram showing a tight LAD lesion (arrow).

The patient underwent angioplasty successfully and had symptom relief on follow-up.

Learning points: Clinicians should be wary of a number of biases that the human mind is prone to. In this case, despite the obvious likelihood of CAD, a preemptive diagnosis of sarcoidosis was presumed and instead of profiling a lesion assiduously, reliance on a recently procured cardiac MRI was considered by the treating team.! Fortunately, a lingering suspicion of incomplete diagnosis persisted that led to a TMT and appropriate management.

Sidelights: What are the common biases you can recall that impact a clinical diagnosis?

Answer: One should be mindful of cognitive, affective, and social biases. The worst is to stereotype a patient's symptoms on racial, gender, or other biases because of the difference in the background of patients. Also important is to be mindful of our own mental state that can over- or underappreciate the issues and the implications thereof. Thus physician's personality determines their risk tolerance and overconfidence, or risk aversion and ambiguity tolerance. The more talked about cognitive biases are confirmation bias (because of a similar recent case), anchoring bias (relying heavily on the first information received, and premature closure of a case), framing effect (the way the information is framed or presented influences the decision), etc. A dose of equanimity is the best antidote to guard against biases as suggested by Sir William Osler. (Read Aequanimitus by Osler.)

CASE

35

Massive Cardiomegaly

"Spoon feeding in the long run teaches us nothing but the shape of the spoon."

—EM Forster

A newborn was admitted in respiratory distress. He was tachycardiac, had weak pulse, and his X-ray is shown in **Figure 1**. The patient was conservatively managed. No operative intervention was done. The other X-ray is of the same patient after 1 year **(Fig. 2)**. What is the likely possibility? What physiological phenomenon might be responsible for such a favorable outcome?

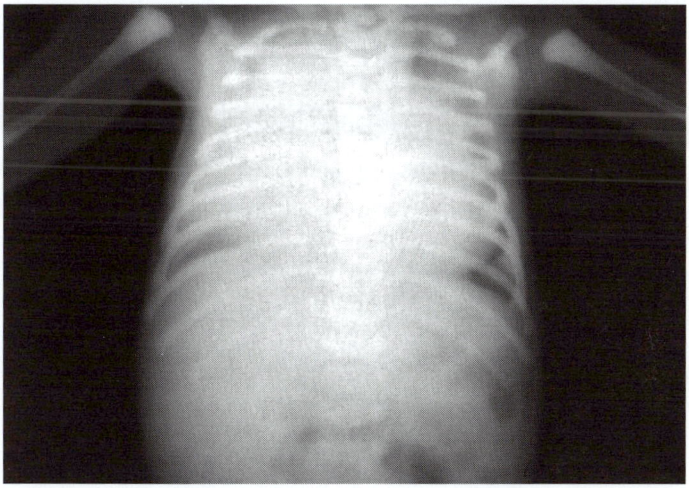

Fig. 1: Chest X-ray of the neonate.

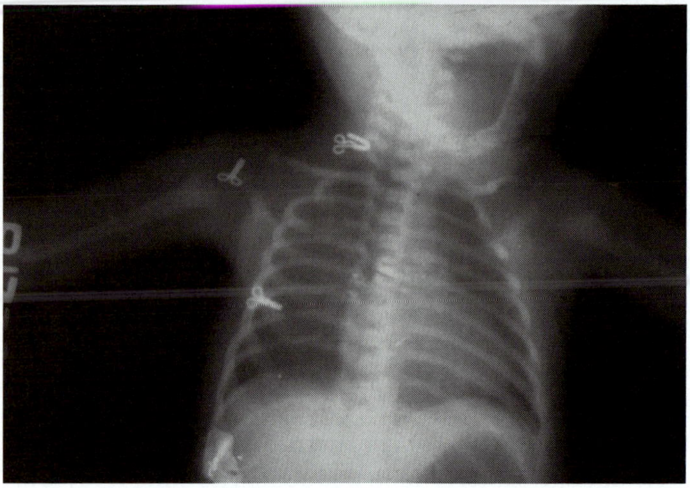

Fig. 2: X-ray of the same patient after 1 year.

Pause and think before you click the answer:

Answer: This is a striking example of an Ebstein anomaly patient whose tricuspid regurgitation (TR) regressed with transition from fetal to adult life. As the pulmonary vascular resistance decreased, the severity of TR also decreased, and finally, the child did not require any intervention for his Ebstein's anomaly. Most neonates with such a severe TR might not be so lucky!

- A 1-and-a-half-year-old child with a similar-looking chest X-ray had a different story **(Fig. 3)**. He had progressively worsening respiratory distress after a normal delivery and at 1 year, the infant was quite breathless at rest. The resting oxymetric saturation was 78%. The patient's echo showed a structurally normal heart.

Unlike Ebstein's anomaly that improves with time in the early neonatal period due to a decrease in pulmonary vascular resistance (PVR), this child progressively worsened. His present X-ray is shown in Figure 3. He had an operative intervention done to get the postoperative X-ray in **Figure 4**. What intervention is likely?

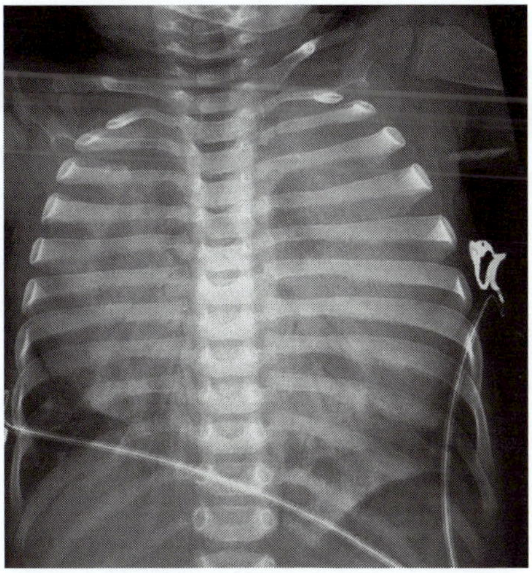

Fig. 3: Preoperative X-ray.

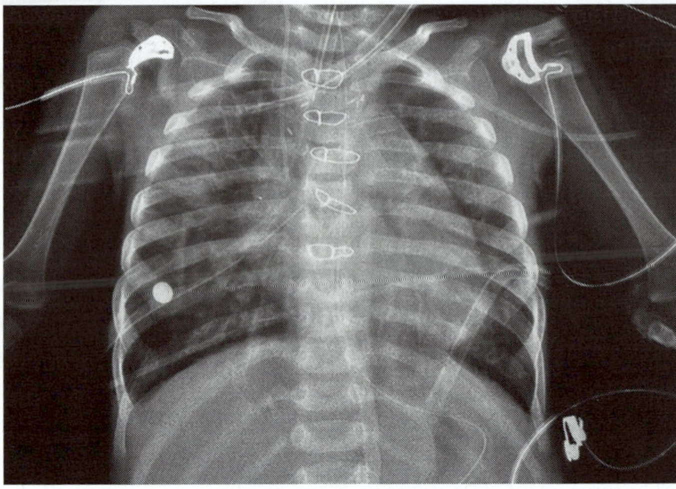

Fig. 4: Postoperative X-ray.

Pause and think before you click the answer:

Answer: This child had a massive thymoma requiring operative intervention as the lung compression by the mass was causing hypoxia.

The computed tomography (CT) images are shown in **Figure 5**.

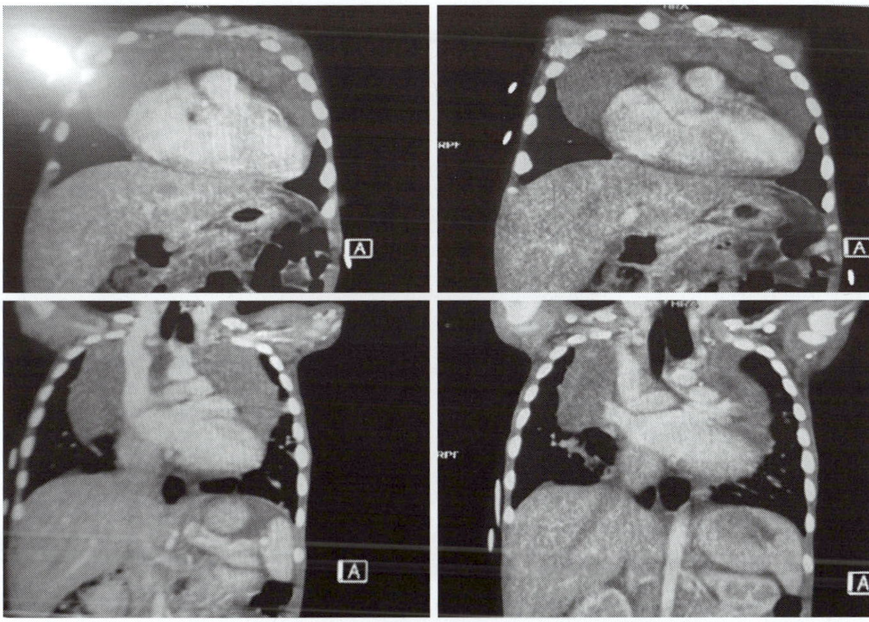

Fig. 5: Computed tomography showing massive thymus.

The resected tumor showed a thymoma. The child recovered completely after the operation. The resected mass is shown in **Figure 6**.

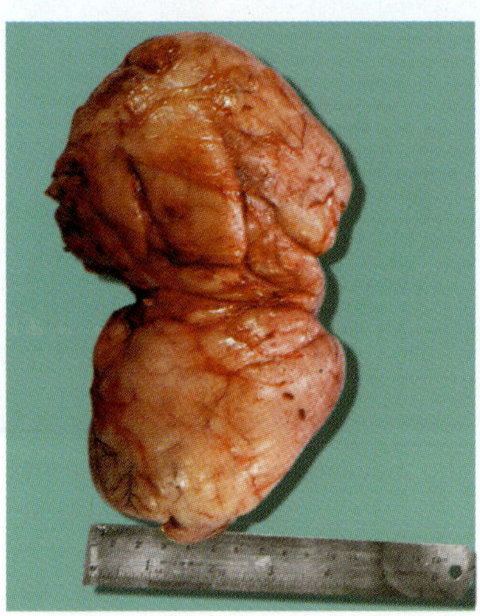

Fig. 6: Thymoma removed.

And yet another cardiomegaly with a normal heart in neonate:

- A 5-day-old newborn had severe respiratory distress since birth. His heart rate was 140 beats/min, respiratory rate 74 breaths/min, and blood pressure was 90/60 mm Hg. The chest X-ray is shown in **Figure 7**.

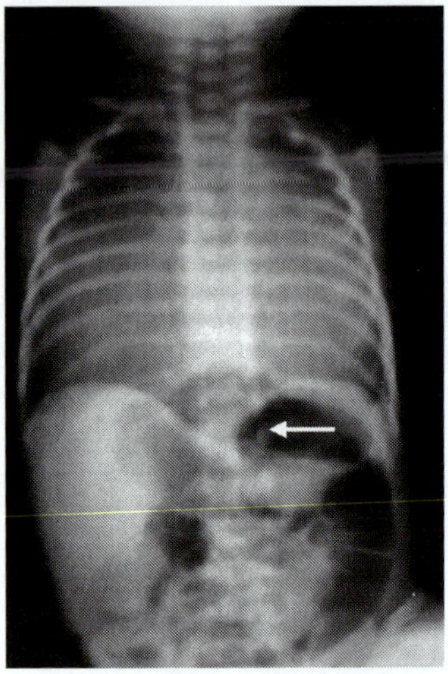

Fig. 7: Chest X-ray of a newborn in distress.

The echo showed a structurally normal heart but with a large pericardial effusion and a mass. The echo is shown in **Figure 8**.

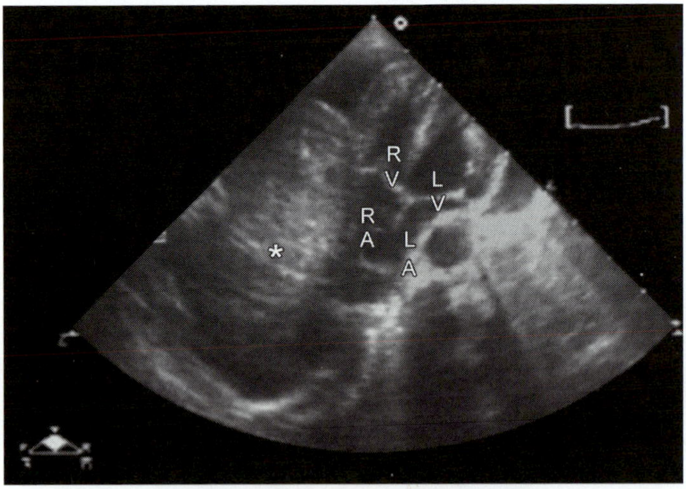

Fig. 8: Echo showing pericardial effusion and a mass.

It was not a pericardial cyst but structurally resembled a liver. The CT is shown in **Figure 9**.

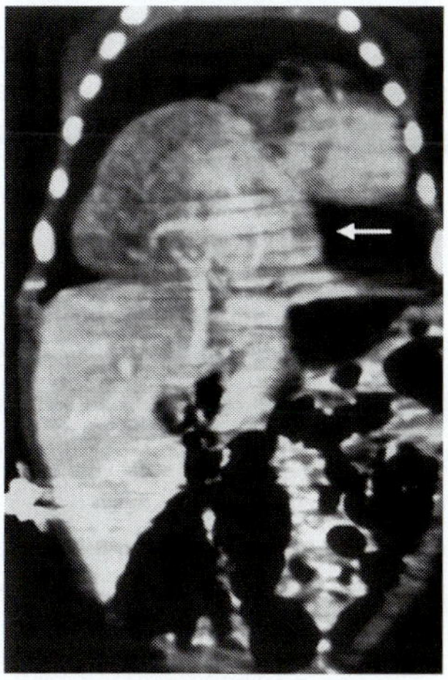

Fig. 9: Computed tomography showing the anatomy.

It was a liver herniation (left lobe of the liver) into the pericardium through a diaphragmatic defect. It is a rare anomaly (presented just for a surprise and to affirm that facts are stranger than fiction.) The child recovered after operative treatment where the hernia was repaired and the liver placed back in the abdomen.

(*Source:* Anandaraja S, Kumar A, Agarwala S, Gulati GS, Bal CS, Kothari SS. Liver herniation into the pericardium: an unusual cause of massive pericardial effusion with intrapericardial mass in a neonate. Pediatr Cardiol. 2005;26(6):862-5.)

Learning points: The impact of transitional circulation on cardiac hemodynamics should be kept in mind in evaluating infants.

Developmental defects need to be considered in neonates.

Sidelights:

1. **What happens if the transitional circulation does not take place?**
2. **Which cardiac disorders may masquerade as persistent pulmonary hypertension of newborn (PPHN)?**

(*Sidelights are food for thought—provided to increase your curiosity:* So as a rule, do not read these answers before you try to answer them yourself. The answers provided here are not intended to be exhaustive.)

Answer: If the transitional circulation does not happen normally, the newborn does not get enough pulmonary blood flow or oxygenation and suffers from serious hypoxemia and its consequences. This usually occurs from disorders such as prematurity and unavailability of surfactants (respiratory distress syndrome), birth asphyxia, meconium aspiration, pulmonary hypoplasia, diaphragmatic hernia, idiopathic PPHN (10% of times of the PPHN), and maternal use of NSAIDs/SSRI in pregnancy. Intensive ventilator efforts with high-frequency ventilators, pulmonary vasodilators, inotropes, surfactants, or ECMO may be required to tide over the crisis till the transitional circulation might take place. With intensive management, mortality might be around 10%.

- While pediatricians are familiar with PPHN, there is a tendency to over diagnose PPHN as echo measurements of PA pressures have become commonplace. Many times, obstructed total anomalous pulmonary venous connection (TAPVC), hypoplastic left heart syndrome, arch obstruction, and hemitruncus/AP window are missed by an amateur echo cardiographer. Hence, a high index of suspicion for cardiac disorders should be kept unless the PPHN is fitting in the clinical context of the newborn.

It is less well realized that in some of the ventricular septal defect (VSD) Eisenmenger syndrome patients that present in adults, there was no past history suggestive of a left to right shunt. In some of them at least, the regression of pulmonary vascular resistance index (PVRI) never occurred and the persistence of high fetal PVRI prevented symptoms usually seen in babies with VSDs. Nor did they have severe hypoxia-like other cases of PPHN!

- Thus, when a 9 months infant with posterior muscular VSD presented with right to left shunt and a saturation of 85%, it was thought that this might be the patient with persistent fetal circulation. He had dilated right ventricle and a pulmonary regurgitation jet suggestive of mean PA pressure of 60 mm Hg.

The echo is shown in **Video 1**.

Video 1

But a moment of inspiration allowed to investigate for something. The video showing the intervention is shown below. Can you understand what is the procedure done after seeing the video **(Video 2)** and the pictures **(Figs. 10 and 11)**?

Video 2

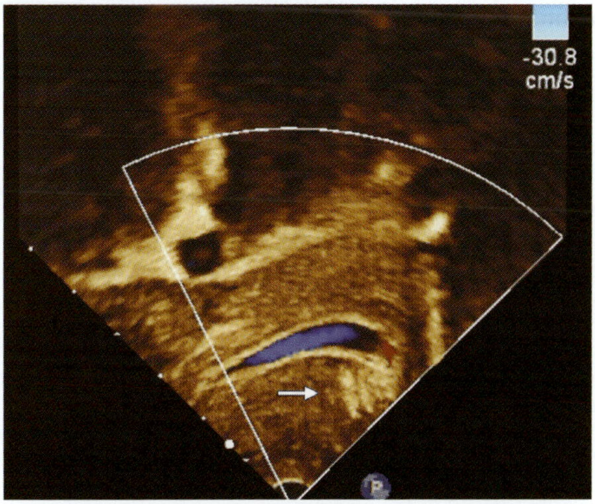

Fig. 10: Liver seen by echo after the procedure.

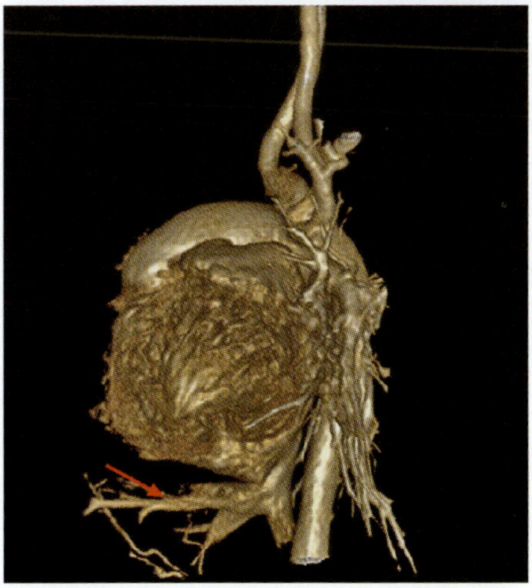

Fig. 11: The CT image is shown (the red arrow).

Answer: The patient had an intrahepatic portosystemic shunt connecting a branch of the left portal vein to the inferior vena cava (IVC) just above the confluence of hepatic vein drainage to IVC as shown by the arrow in Figure 11. The anomalous branch was closed by a vascular plug. (white arrow). (Video 2).! We hope that PA pressure would reduce and patient is not in Eisenmenger state. The patient is being followed up.

CASE

36

Hiccups in the Diagnosis

"No matter what you look at, if you look at it closely enough, you are involved in the entire universe."

—Michael Faraday

A 50-year-old previously healthy executive had persistent hiccups lasting for 3 days. There was no history of chest pain, fever, dietary indiscretion, alcohol intake, or any other obvious stressors. The blood pressure was once recorded as 190/100 mm Hg during the hiccups, but all other readings were within normal range. Physical examination was unremarkable. Routine investigations including troponins were within normal limits. The ECG and chest X-ray are shown in **Figures 1 and 2**. The hiccups settled down after 3 days, but the patient had an episode of transient loss of consciousness and hence was referred. The ECG showed no regional wall motion abnormality. The troponins were normal again. The echo is shown below. A 24-hour holter did not show any abnormality. Heart rate varied from 65 to 100 beats/min. An ambulatory blood pressure recording did not show hypertension. Mean systolic and diastolic pressures were recorded as 115/72 mm Hg. The patient had another witnessed episode of brief loss of consciousness as he sat down after straining at stools lasting for less than a minute. A coronary angio with intravascular ultrasound (IVUS) showed plaque in the left anterior descending artery (LAD) with 60% lumen loss.

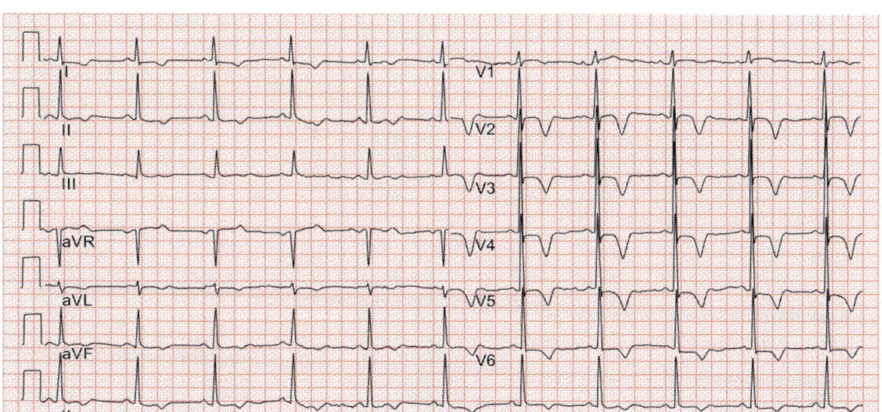

Fig. 1: ECG.

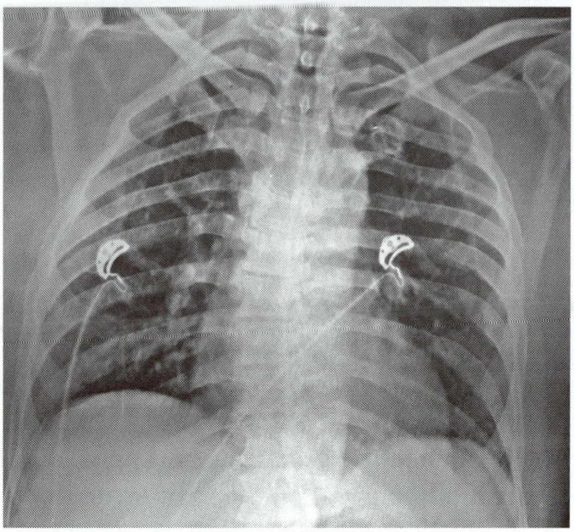

Fig. 2: Chest X-ray.

*Echocardiogram **(Video 1)**:*

Video 1

The coronary angiogram and IVUS are shown here ***(Videos 2 and 3)***:

Video 2 **Video 3**

The IVUS at the lesion showed around 60% lumen loss and a stable plaque **(Fig. 3)**.

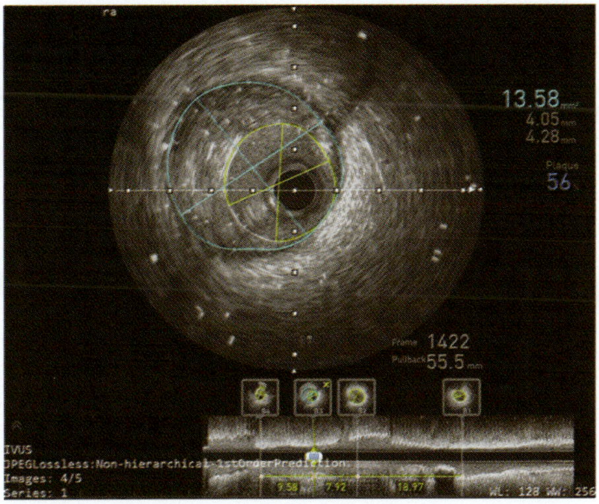

Fig. 3: Intravascular ultrasound (IVUS) showing luminal narrowing of approximately 60%.

Blood sugar during the episode was normal. Serum metanephrine and tryptase were normal.

Should we stent the LAD?

The ECG in a nonhypertensive patient was suggestive of hypertrophic cardiomyopathy (HCM). A magnetic resonance imaging (MRI) (and ECHO) showed apical hypertrophic cardiomyopathy. The patient had another episode of brief loss of consciousness with perspiration while straining at the stool while the holter was attached. The holter recording showed only sinus bradycardia. One EEG done when the patient had no symptoms was normal.

A brain MRI showed recent infarcts in different vascular territories.

What is the diagnosis?

Pause and think before you click the answer:

Answer: The patient had cardioembolic stroke, causing hiccups and also episodic syncope from dysautonomia. Hiccups can occur from numerous causes, but hiccups due to a cerebrovascular accident (CVA) are less well recognized. The episodes of syncope were too brief and self-limiting and luckily, we identified sinus bradycardia during one of the episodes. In the real world, such patients could have received percutaneous transluminal coronary angioplasty (PTCA) to LAD (and then ticagrelor-induced bradycardia as the diagnosis of syncope, or an implantable cardioverter defibrillator (ICD) due to apical hypertrophic cardiomyopathy syncope).

Sinus bradycardia or sinus arrest due to dysautonomia following a CVA is also less recognized. Such episodes have been reported with brain stem or occipital lobe infarcts. Acute lacunar infarct in this patient is shown in **Figures 4A to G** that could result in autonomic dysfunction. The patient's episodes did not recur, and he was on anticoagulation and statins with aspirin for stable CAD, thus affirming the impression that CVA was the cause of dysautonomia. The patient was not on any medication that could cause sinus bradycardia.

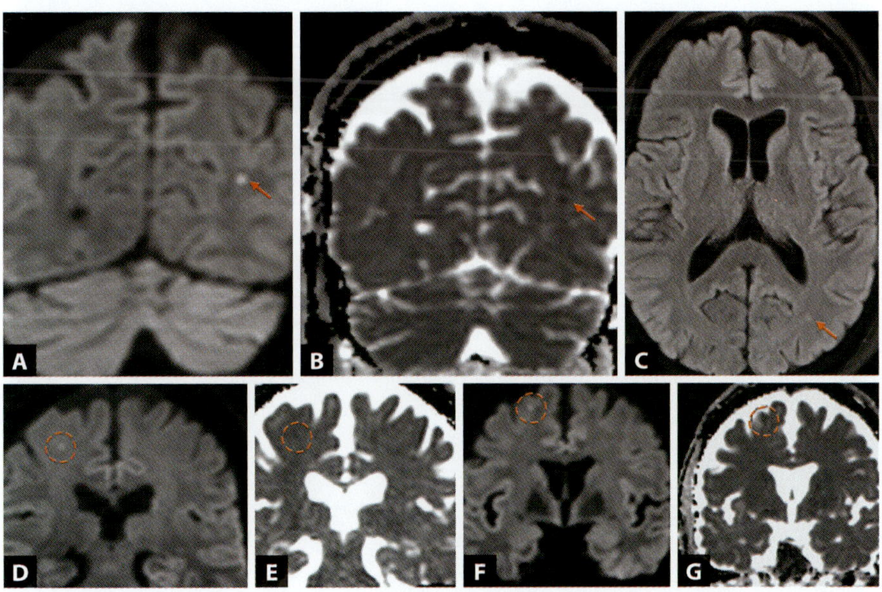

Figs. 4A to G: MRI brain (3 tesla scanner). Diffusion-weighted (b-1000) axial image (A) and the corresponding ADC map (B) shows a tiny focus of diffusion restriction in the subcortical white matter of left posterior parieto-occipital junction (arrow) with FLAIR (C) hyperintense signal intensity suggestive of a tiny acute infarct. A few other tiny foci of diffusion restriction were also noted in the right frontal lobe (dashed circle) (D to G), b-1000 (D and F) and corresponding ADC map (E and G). Tiny infarcts in multiple vascular territories were noted raising the possibility of cardioembolic origin.

Learning points: Apical hypertrophic cardiomyopathy might be missed, but a deep T-wave inversion and left ventricular hypertrophy (especially in the absence of severe hypertension) should alert the physician. It might be a cause of cardioembolic stroke.

Hiccups and sinus arrests could occur from posterior circulation stroke.

A plaque in LAD might be a bystander!

Sidelights: When "hypertrophic cardiomyopathy" is not hypertrophic cardiomyopathy?

Answer: The echocardiographic phenotype of HCM might be simulated by other clinical conditions, that is the point of the question. Athlete heart, hypertensive heart disease, and cardiac amyloidosis are commonly considered differential diagnosis for HCM. But in atypical HCM, Fabry's disease, glycogen storage disease (Pompe's disease), mitochondrial myopathies, infiltrative disorders, and rarely sarcoidosis also need to be considered.

Mostly, the distinction is obvious once the possibilities are kept in the mind. Typically, this non-HCM masqueraders do not exhibit high contractility typically seen in HCM. There might be heart failure which is not seen in HCM until late, or other systemic symptoms that might give away the clue. Remember, burning hands and feet, lack of excessive perspiration, and cutaneous angiomas as the indicators for Fabry's disease (but HCM-like heart could present in the absence of these), a generalized weakness for adult onset Pompe's disease; and other system involvement for mitochondrial myopathies like myopathy, lactic acidosis and sideroblastic anemia (MLASA) should be the clues to the right diagnosis.

- But here is an adult patient with HCM and markedly elevated jugular venous pressure (JVP). He did not have any of the above entities. Nor was his left ventricular (LV) function too poor. Why was there so much heart failure? The echo is shown here **(Videos 4 to 7)**.

Video 4 Video 5 Video 6 Video 7

Answer: Severe right ventricular (RV) hypertrophy in patients with HCM might cause heart failure with RV diastolic and systolic dysfunction. This patient's cardiac cath revealed a right atrial pressure of 22 mm Hg. MRI revealed hypertrophic cardiomyopathy and extensive muscle bundles in RV as well. However, still the RA mean of 22 mm Hg appeared unusual. There were multiple mediastinal lymph nodes and constitutional features suggestive of tuberculosis. Whether there was associated constrictive pericarditis with HCM accounting for heart failure remained unproven but very likely, even though the pericardium was not thickened on MRI!

CASE

37

More of Mitral Stenosis

"The journey of a thousand miles begins with a single step."

—Lao Tzu

A 20-year-old man with dyspnea and congestive heart failure had severe mitral stenosis with a valve area of 1 cm^2 on 2D echo. His cath pressure tracings are shown in **Figure 1**.

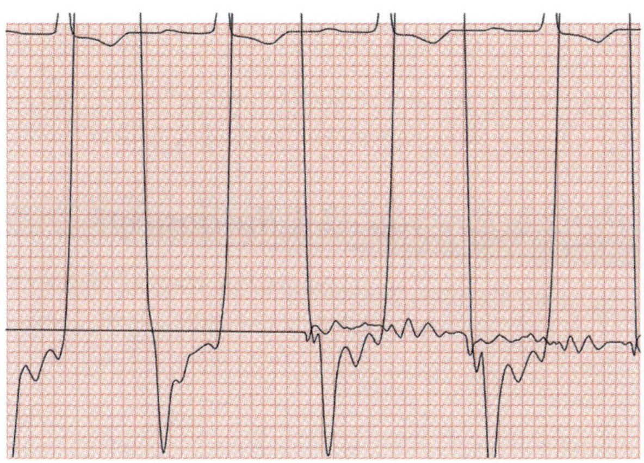

Fig. 1: Pulmonary artery wedge (PAW) and left ventricular (LV) pressure tracings.

The tracings of LV and PAW show minimal end diastolic gradients. Why? What are the possible reasons?

Pause and think before you click the answer:

Answer: The tracings show small gradients despite a severe mitral stenosis on echo. An unreliable wedge pressure is not uncommon due to wedging in the walls, so first one should ensure that the wedge pressure trace is reliable. Long cycles in atrial fibrillation (AF), or bradycardia in a patient might lead to a lack of end-diastolic gradients. Gradients are related to output, so very poor cardiac output can proportionately reduce gradients. However, in this patient, those arguments do not seem to account for the lack of a significant gradient. The detailed hemodynamic data are shown in **Table 1**.

TABLE 1: Hemodynamic data.

Chamber	*Sys (v)*	*Dias (a)*	*Mean*	*O_2%*
SVC				43.2
RA	13	11	12	90
PA	85	25	50	91.7
PV	14	15	14	97.0
LA			14	
LVED	125	14		
AO	125	80	95	96.0

(AO: aorta; LA: left atrium; LVED: left ventricular end-diastolic; PA: pulmonary artery; PV: pulmonary vein; RA: right atrium; SVC: superior vena cava)

The diagnosis is obvious after seeing the data that the patient has Lutembacher syndrome [atrial septal defect (ASD) and mitral stenosis].

The question is how sick is this patient?

Pause and think before you click the answer:

Answer: A mixed venous saturation of 43% indicates very low cardiac output and hence a very sick patient.

- Another 50-year-old man with rheumatic mitral stenosis who had undergone a closed mitral valvotomy 20 years back presented with a recurrence of symptoms and heart failure. His ECG and chest X-ray are shown in **Figures 2 and 3**.

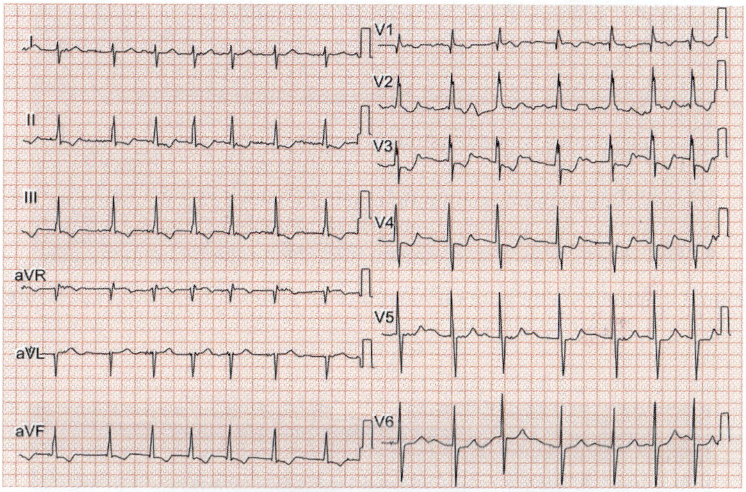

Fig. 2: ECG.

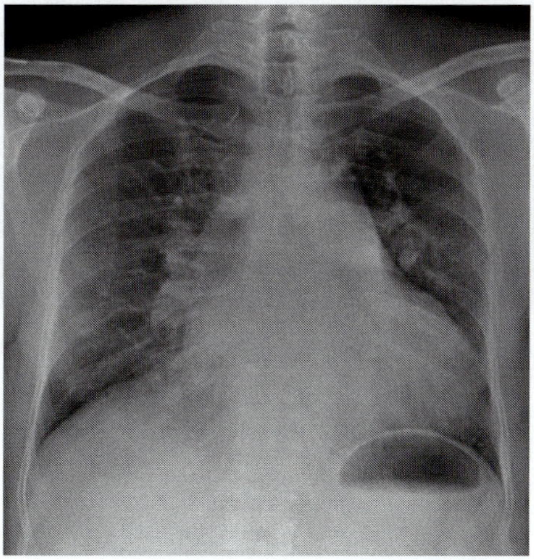

Fig. 3: Chest X-ray.

He underwent a cardiac catheterization, and his left ventricle and PAW pressure tracings are shown in **Figures 4 and 5**.

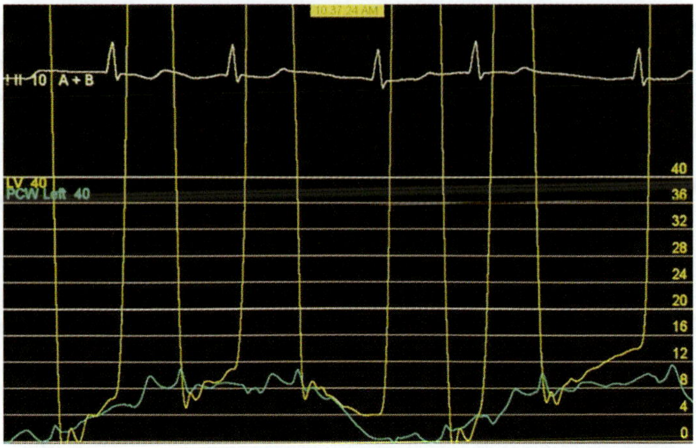

Fig. 4: Left pulmonary artery (PA) wedge and left ventricular (LV) pressure.

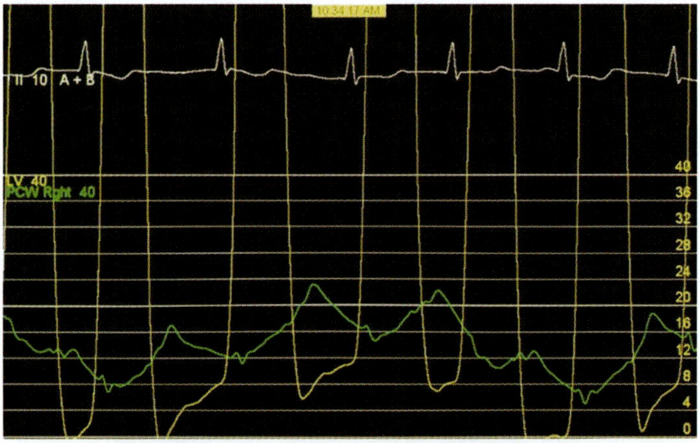

Fig. 5: Right pulmonary artery (PA) wedge and left ventricular (LV) pressure.

Why there is a difference in gradients on the two sides?

Pause and think before you click the answer:

Answer: The wedge pressures in different zones of the lungs might be slightly different. But the tracings and differences in this case seem more than that. Does the chest X-ray give you any clue? If not, have a close look at the angiograms below. The picture is not very good, but see it carefully **(Videos 1 to 3)**.

Video 1 **Video 2** **Video 3**

The patient's hemodynamic data are given in **Table 2**. Rehearse this to identify the problem. It is quite obvious by now, though.

TABLE 2: CATH data of a 50-year-old mitral stenosis patient.

CATH data Hb: 13.2 g/dL; ABG-pH: 7.4; pO_2: 94 mm; HCO_3: 25 mEq/L; SaO_2: 97%			
	Saturation (%)		***Pressures (mm Hg)***
RIJV	61		
Left vertical vein	89		
Left innominate vein	86	SVC	V15 m9
Rt subclavian vein	84	CS	V12 m 9
High SVC	74	RA	V12 m9
Low SVC	73	RV	50 ed 12
IVC	73	RPA wedge	V22 m 18
RA	74	LPA wedge	V12 m 8
Coronary sinus	90	LV	120 ed 8
Pulmonary artery	72	AO	120/70
Left lower pulmonary vein	99		
Femoral artery	97		

(AO: aorta; CS: coronary sinus; IVC: inferior vena cava; LPA: left pulmonary artery; LV: left ventricle; RA: right atrium; RIJV: right internal jugular vein; RPA: right pulmonary artery; RV: right ventricle; SVC: superior vena cava)

The patient had a partial anomalous pulmonary venous connection (PAPVC) with mitral stenosis (MS). The chest X-ray did show pulmonary vascularity increased on the left side. The left-sided veins are draining anomalously to the coronary sinus and left innominate vein. The contrasting clinical findings in ASD with MS and in PAPVC with MS are very interesting.

In ASD with MS, it is the MS that is missed on clinical examination and the patient appears to be a case of an ASD with a large shunt and heart failure; whereas in PAPVC with MS, it is the PAPVC that is missed on examination and findings of MS are dominant. PAPVC with MS is quite rarely seen but makes an interesting hemodynamic puzzle in the sense that pulmonary flows in two lungs are different—the flow in the anomalous PAPVC side has increased blood flow.

Now that we are on the tracings of mitral stenosis, shown below is the tracing of a patient with severe MS and no ASD **(Fig. 6)**. The gradient is varying and abolished even despite MS. What might be the reason for it?

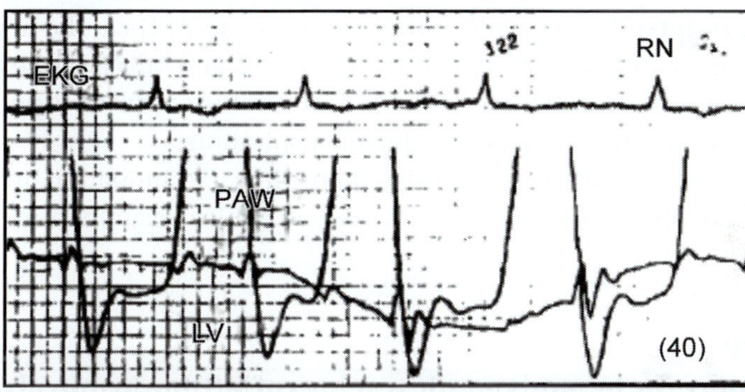

Fig. 6: PA wedge and LV pressure tracing in yet another patient with mitral stenosis.

Pause and think before you click the answer:

Answer: The patient had constrictive pericarditis and mitral stenosis. During inspiration, the PAW pressure would decrease due to the intrathoracic location of the lungs, but the decrease is not reflected in the LVEDP as it is encased in a thick pericardium resulting in changes with respiration. The mechanism is analogous to more known ventricular interdependence.

(*Source:* Kothari SS, Narula J, Tandon R, Shrivastava S. Cardiac compression with mitral stenosis: a haemodynamic challenge. Int J Cardiol. 1993;39(3): 216-8.)

Learning points: Patients with mitral stenosis and ASD can have minimal gradients at the mitral valve. Patients with PAPVC and MS can have different gradients on two sides. Patients with MS and chronic constrictive pericarditis (CCP) may have a reverse gradient during inspiration.

In ASD and MS, MS might be missed on clinical examination. In patients of PAPVC and MS, PAPVC might be missed on clinical examination.

Sidelights:

1. **Compare the hemodynamic tracings of MS due to mitral annular calcium and MS due to rheumatic heart disease (RHD).**
2. **Is there LV dysfunction in MS?**

(*Sidelights are food for thought—provided to increase your curiosity:* So as a rule, do not read these answers before you try to answer them yourself. The answers provided here are not intended to be exhaustive.)

Answer: There is a true obstruction to inflow in RHD MS patients and the Y wave is blunted, whereas the patients with mitral annular calcium (MAC) have a rapid Y wave due to increased mean LA pressure from the associated LV diastolic dysfunction and/or heart failure with preserved ejection fraction (HFpEF). Thus, elevated mean LA pressure does not reflect MS severity in MAC in contrast to RHD MS. Valve impedance is low in MAC compared to RHD MS. Thus, for the same degree of LA pressures, balloon mitral valvuloplasty (BMV) may be very helpful to RHD MS whereas transcatheter mitral valve replacement (TMVR) may not be as helpful in MAC to relieve the symptoms.

(*Source:* Reddy YNV. Complexity of Defining Severe "Stenosis" From Mitral Annular Calcification. Circulation. 2019;140(7):523-5.)

- Left ventricular dysfunction in MS is sometimes present and is attributed to disuse atrophy, as chronic preload deprivation might cause contractile dysfunction in the long term. Oftentimes, tachycardiomyopathy from the associated AF would be the cause. There does not seem to be enough evidence supporting a rheumatic fever-induced myocardial damage by itself.

CASE

38

More of Pulmonary Arterial Hypertension

"Lead me from the unreal to the real. Lead me from darkness to light. Lead me from death to immortality."

—The Upanishads

An 18-year-old girl presented with worsening breathlessness and anemia for the last 2 years. The patient required blood transfusion multiple times with hemoglobin dropping to 6–7 g% in the last 2 years. Hematologic evaluation revealed sideroblastic anemia. She was referred to cardiology services because her breathlessness persisted despite a blood transfusion and hemoglobin of 11 g%.

At presentation, the patient was dyspneic, with tachycardia, and systemic desaturation. Her arterial blood gases showed pH 7.46, pO_2 46 mm Hg, pCO_2 38 mm Hg, and serum lactate 2.5 mmol/L. The serum electrolytes and renal and liver functions were normal except for the serum bilirubin of 2.5 mg/dL. The ECG, chest X-ray, and echo are shown in **Figures 1 and 2, Videos 1 and 2**.

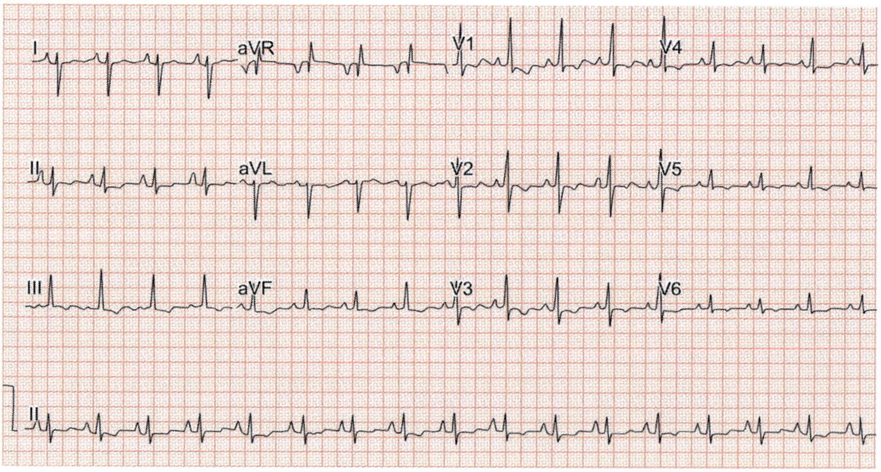

Fig. 1: ECG showing severe right ventricular hypertrophy (RVH).

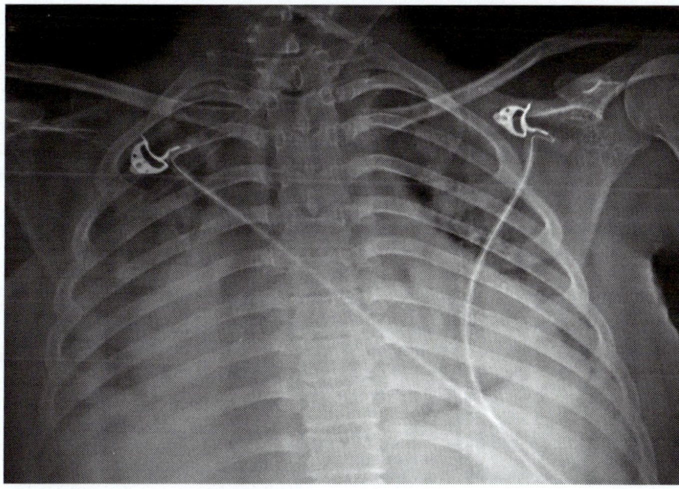

Fig. 2: Portable chest X-ray.

Video 1 **Video 2**

Subsequently, she underwent a cardiac CT and a cardiac catheterization that confirmed the findings of severe pulmonary arterial hypertension (PAH) **(Figs. 3 and 4)**.

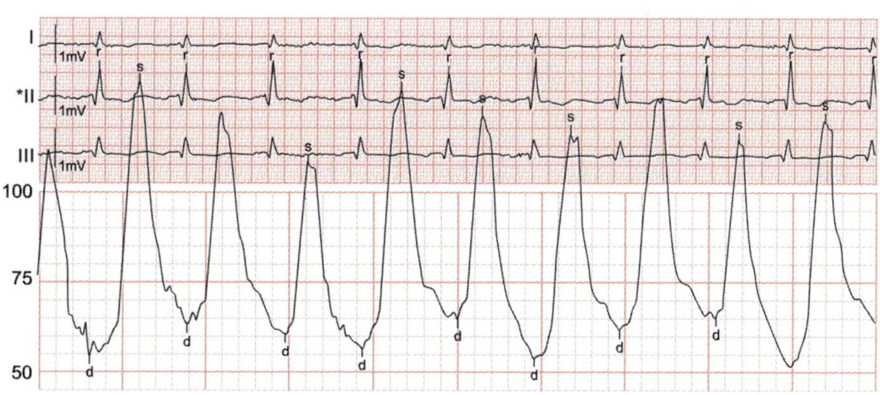

Fig. 3: Pulmonary artery (PA) pressures (114/58 mm Hg) on room air.

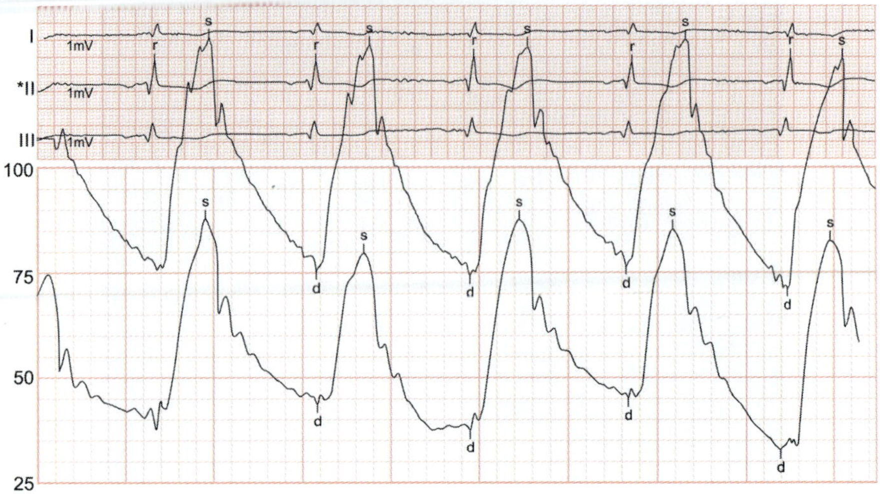

Fig. 4: Pulmonary artery (PA) pressure 83/39(54) and aortic pressure 126/74(96) on 100% oxygen.

Her contrast-enhanced computed tomography (CECT) ***(Videos 3 and 4)****:*

Video 3 **Video 4**

What do you think is the cause of PAH?

Pause and think before you click the answer:

Answer: The patient had congenital sideroblastic anemia from a mitochondrial mutation that is part of myopathy, lactic acidosis, and sideroblastic anemia (MLASA) syndrome. Pulmonary hypertension in hemolytic anemia that causes intravascular hemolysis and ineffective erythropoiesis is well recognized as in sickle cell anemia, β-thalassemia, paroxysmal nocturnal hemoglobinuria, and other congenital dyserythropoietic anemias. The mechanisms of PAH are multiple and include nitric oxide deficiency from the intravascular hemolysis (since hemoglobin mops up nitric oxide), vascular injury from hemolysis-induced release of adenosinc deaminase, and arginase from red blood cells and postcapillary pulmonary hypertension from left ventricular dysfunction due to iron overload and high output from anemia. Even so, such severe PAH was unusual. On genetic analysis, she was found to have a mitochondrial mutation in the *PUS1* gene. We hypothesized that severe PAH might be related to the genetic defect in addition to other causes of hemolytic anemia as above.

A cardiac magnetic resonance imaging (MRI) showed mild iron overload in the liver, but there was no obvious myocardial iron overload **(Fig. 5)**. Cardiac catheterization documented severe PAH with pulmonary artery pressures of 114/58(78) mm Hg and aortic pressure of 120/75(96) mm Hg (Fig. 4). On 100% oxygen with a mask, the PA pressures dropped to 83/40(54) mm Hg. The left ventricular end-diastolic pressure (LVEDP) was 10 mm Hg, and the right atrial pressure was 14 mm Hg. The calculated pulmonary vascular resistance index (PVRI) was 19 wood units.mm^2 on room air that dropped to 12 wood units on oxygen. Vasoreactivity testing with nitric oxide was not done due to nonavailability, but the PA pressures were responsive to oxygen. The patient was treated with pulmonary vasodilator therapy with ambrisentan,

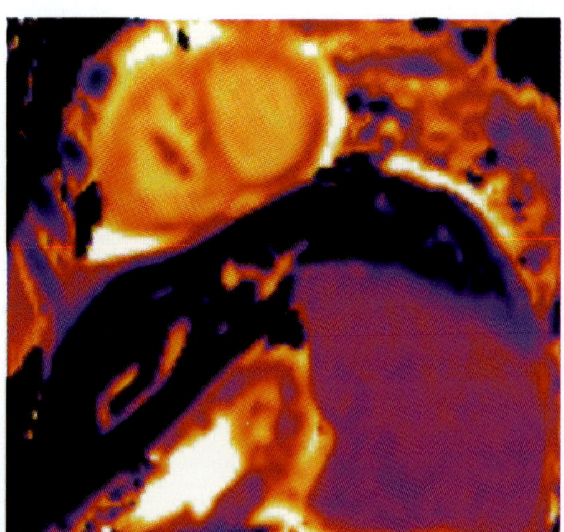

Fig. 5: Magnetic resonance imaging (MRI) showing liver siderosis.

tadalafil, and amlodipine (in view of oxygen responsiveness). She continued to be symptomatic requiring low flow oxygen to maintain oxygen saturation. The oxygen saturation on room air would drop to 75–84% without any hypercarbia. Her transfusion requirements were intermittent, and empirical treatment with pyridoxine and danazol did not change it remarkably. The patient was evaluated for a bone marrow and lung transplant, but the family declined the same.

Learning points: Hemolytic anemia with intravascular hemolysis develops PAH due to multiple causes. Hemoglobin mops up nitric oxide resulting in nitric oxide deficiency and PAH, and arginine liberated from RBCs may be vasculotoxic amongst other factors resulting in PAH.

Sidelights:

1. **What is the utility of the diffusing capacity of the lungs for carbon monoxide (DLCO) in the investigations for PAH?**
2. **Why uric acid is elevated in PAH?**

(*Sidelights are food for thought—provided to increase your curiosity:* So as a rule, do not read these answers before you try to answer them yourself. The answers provided here are not intended to be exhaustive.)

Answer: DLCO (diffusion capacity for carbon monoxide) assesses gas exchange. It is usually reduced in intrinsic lung diseases, such as emphysema, interstitial lung disease, or pulmonary vascular disease. In the absence of evidence of significant pulmonary restrictive or obstructive disease, a reduced DLCO suggests a pulmonary vascular disease such as idiopathic pulmonary hypertension (IPH) or thromboembolic PAH. In pulmonary vascular disease, DLCO is reduced due to impairment of gas exchange at the alveolar-capillary interface. It should be remembered that DLCO is increased in pulmonary hemorrhage, pulmonary edema, and left to right shunts. DLCO 60–74% predicted (Z-score: –1.6 to –2.5) suggest mild impairment, DLCO 40–60% predicted (Z-score: –2.5 to –4) moderate impairment, and DLCO values <40% predicted (Z-score: <–4) suggest severe impairment.

- Uric acid is elevated in patients with PAH and is a prognostic marker. The raised levels might result from decreased renal perfusion, decreased pulmonary blood flow, or altered purine metabolisms in the diseased remodeling pulmonary vasculature. Whether it may be a therapeutic target in influencing the disease progression is being actively investigated.

CASE

39

Hypertension and Lung Disease

"Talent perceives differences; genius, unity."

—WB Yeats

A 36-year-old man presented with history of progressive breathlessness and fatigue for last 2 years. The patient was accustomed to heavy manual work and he has worked as a stone cutter for few years. He did not have any significant illness previously, and there was no family history of hypertension or sudden death. On examination, he had severe hypertension 180/110 mm Hg, mild aortic regurgitation and scattered rhonchi. The routine investigations were normal except a raised creatinine 1.5 mg%. His X-ray and ECG are shown in **Figures 1 and 2**.

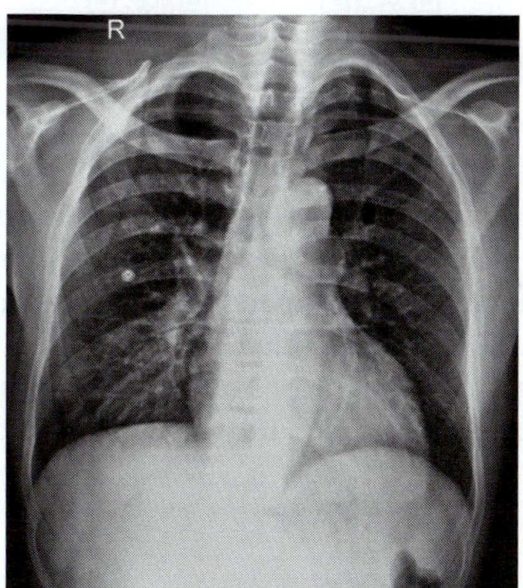

Fig. 1: Chest X-ray showing prominent aorta, LV configuration of apex and calcified spots in the hilar region (*see* CT).

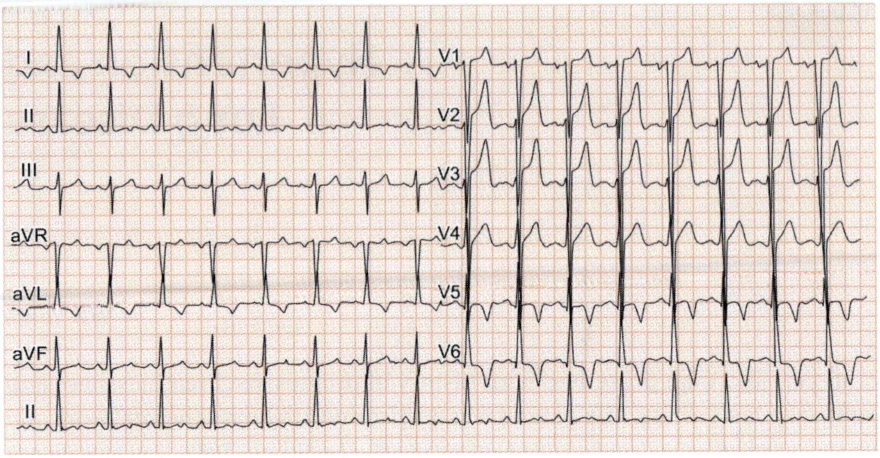

Fig. 2: ECG showing left ventricular hypertrophy (LVH) with strain.

The echo showed left ventricular hypertrophy and mildly reduced ejection fraction (EF) with mild AR **(Videos 1 and 2)**.

Video 1 **Video 2**

The pulmonary function tests (PFTs) revealed reduced vital capacity (70% of predicted), decrease forced expiratory volume in the first second (FEV1) (79% of predicted), and reduced diffusing capacity of the lungs for carbon monoxide (DLCO) (67% predicted).

The renal ultrasound showed normal-sized kidneys with maintained corticomedullary differentiation and no evidence of renal artery stenosis.

The patient had severe hypertension, mild kidney disease, restrictive lung disease, and severe left ventricular hypertrophy. His CT scan is shown below that showed calcified lymph nodes suggestive of egg shell calcification **(Figs. 3A and B)**.

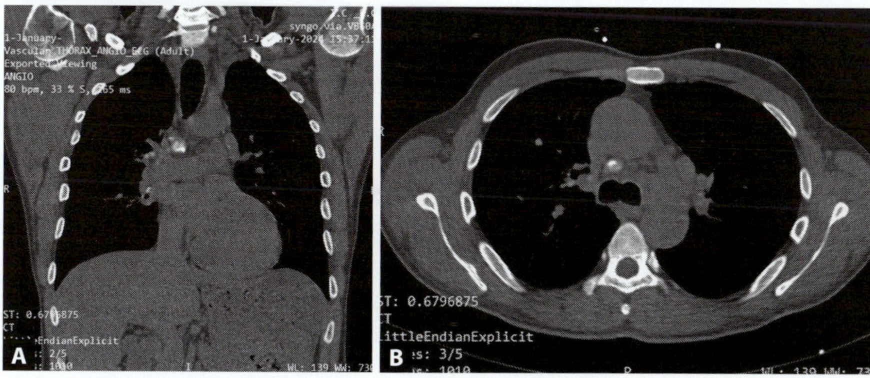

Figs. 3A and B: Coronal (A), and transverse section (B) of cardiac CT showing calcification in the lymph nodes.

What are the possibilities?

Pause and think before you click the answer:

Answer: The case is presented to bring out two important points:

- The constellation of findings in a person who has worked as a stone cutter should bring to mind the possibilities of silicosis. The eggshell calcification, PFT findings, and hypertension are quite compatible with the diagnosis. It is imperative on the physician that the patient's working environment and his occupation should be considered while trying to find a diagnosis; alas, it is often neglected.

  Further, it is not recognized that kidney disease and hypertension also result from silicosis. The mechanisms of hypertension and kidney disease in silicosis are varied and not well understood. The patient had a heavy silicosis exposure and the diagnosis appear very likely. With this lymph node pictures, tuberculosis and sarcoidosis need be considered as well (silicosis patients are also prone to develop tuberculosis or sarcoid), but there was nothing else suggestive for the same.
- Whether the patient has hypertensive heart disease or hypertrophic cardiomyopathy (HCM) is not clear. How to distinguish hypertensive heart from HCM?

  The magnitude of hypertrophy or the site of hypertrophy does not distinguish the two. Genetic testing might help. More recently, MRI showing typical late gadolinium enhancement (LGE) of HCM, or increase in T1 values might favor HCM, although late stages of hypertensive heart disease can also have LGE. This patients MRI is shown in **Figure 4**. The T1 values on MRI were mildly elevated. Further, there are not many reports of MRI in patients with silicosis, so that is an additional problem in distinguishing the two entities in this patient.

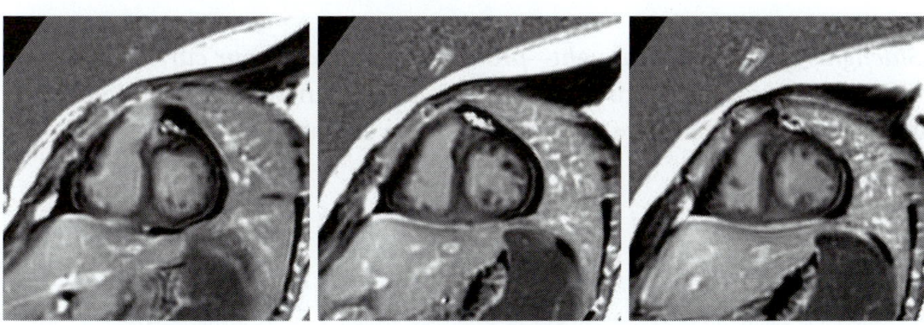

Fig. 4: MRI did not suggest HCM.

Further, a myocardial biopsy was done for the distinction. It showed interstitial fibrosis consistent with hypertensive heart disease and did not suggest HCM **(Figs. 5A and B)**.

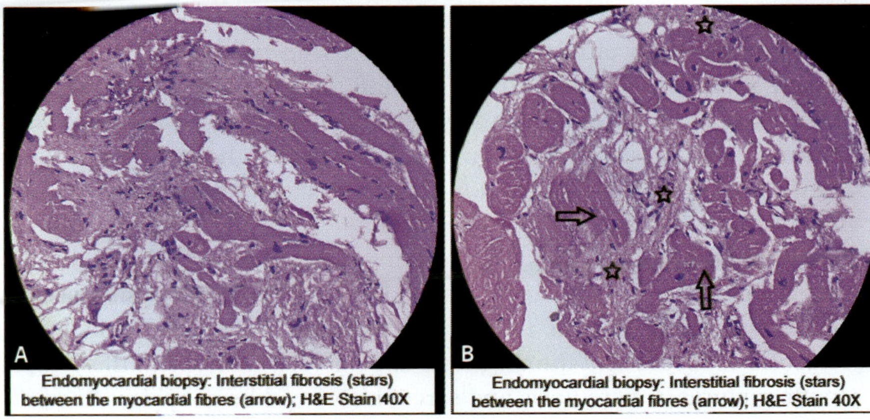

Figs. 5A and B: Myocardial biopsy showing interstitial fibrosis consistent with hypertensive heart failure.

Learning points: Silicosis can cause hypertension, in addition to well-known pulmonary complications.

Patients occupational history can sometimes provide very important clues to the diagnosis.

Sidelights: What are the other causes of occupational exposure resulting in atherosclerosis?

(*Sidelights are food for thought—provided to increase your curiosity:* So as a rule, do not read these answers before you try to answer them yourself. The answers provided here are not intended to be exhaustive.)

Answer: Epidemiological studies have shown association of heavy metal levels in the body and atherosclerosis including arsenic, copper, lead, mercury, and cadmium. Thus the occupation involving these might result in increased atherosclerosis. Such exposure might occur in smelting, mining, and other industrial activities. Exposure to polychlorinated biphenyls (PCB) in the environment may accelerate atherosclerosis (as found in frequent consumers of fish in the areas with high PCB contents in fish.) Environmental pollution and atherosclerosis is an area of intense research focus currently. Polycyclic aromatic hydrocarbons formed by incomplete combustion of organic matter, PCBs, heavy metals, pesticides, and other toxins might be responsible, in part, for the epidemic of atherosclerosis. Occupational details should be investigated in the clinical context.

CASE

40

Total Anomalous Pulmonary Venous Connection Unplugged

"You must be the change you wish to see in the world."

—Mahatma Gandhi

A 7-month-old child was brought to the outpatient department services for the evaluation of feeding difficulty and failure to thrive, and mild cyanosis. The chest X-ray showed typical figure of 8 and pulmonary plethora **(Fig. 1)**. A typical supracardiac total anomalous pulmonary venous connection (TAPVC) with moderate pulmonary arterial hypertension (PAH) was found on echocardiography. The atrial septal defect (ASD) was adequate. The patient elected to come for operation after few months for logistic reasons.

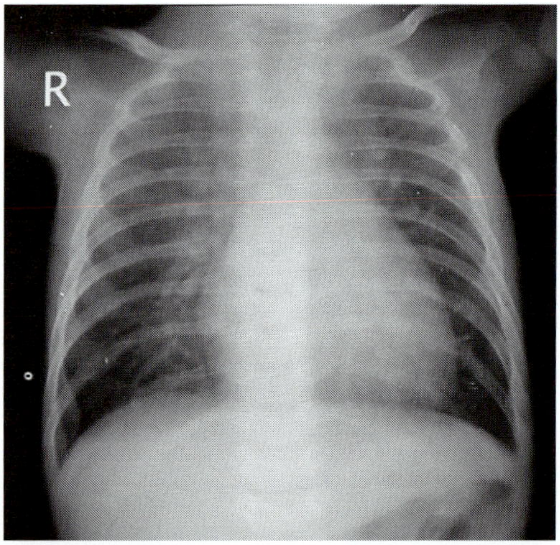

Fig. 1: Chest X-ray consistent with supracardiac total anomalous pulmonary venous connection (TAPVC).

After 2 weeks, the patient was brought to the emergency services with significant worsening of breathlessness. The mother reported that the baby was well few hours prior and as she came back from some routine chores, the child appeared breathless.

What are the reasons for deterioration in a TAPVC? And what possibly in this child? A repeat chest X-ray is shown in **Figure 2**.

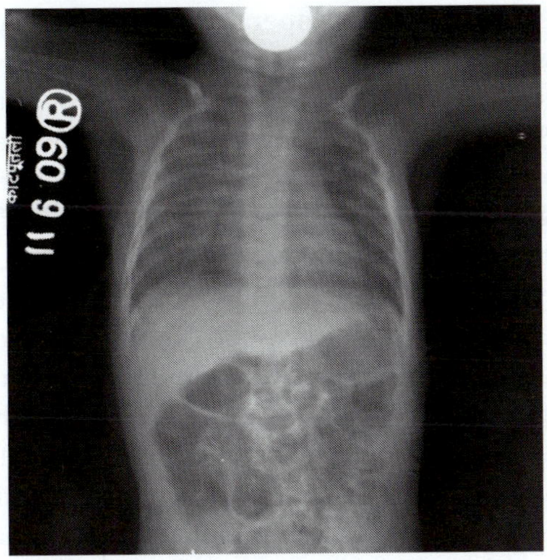

Fig. 2: Chest X-ray of the same child with total anomalous pulmonary venous connection (TAPVC) and distress.

Pause and think before you click the answer:

Answer: The TAPVC generally is operated whenever diagnosed as the heart failure can worsen in infancy, although some patients with TAPVC and an adequate ASD can survive long as adults. The repeat echo did not show worsening of ASD or PAH. The ASD was adequate. Sometimes, a restrictive ASD might become more restrictive while waiting for operation and a balloon septostomy can improve the clinical status in these infants, if immediate operation is not possible. The child appeared in distress. The X-ray shows a coin in the pharynx that the baby somehow ingested while mother was away. A prompt bronchoscopy and foreign body removal cured the problem. The infant was operated for TAPVC with no further ado. It is important that we do not disregard the history (the distress worsened suddenly while the mother was away..!), and keep common sense still intact in the AI era. No cardiology resident thought about the coin in this case! (overspecialization may lead to extinction of the species, if the environment suddenly changes).

Learning points: Common sense is not common, but should be consciously cultivated as much as possible, more so if you specialize.

Sidelights: Recapitulate similar incidences in your practice. This introspection will teach, if internalized.

The next 10 cases (case 41–50) actually need a pertinent sharp observation or an idea only; they are short snippets. The learning point is obvious after the answer.

CASE

41

Cyanosis

"The real voyage of discovery consists not in seeking new lands, but in seeing with new eyes."

—Marcel Proust

A 4-year-old had cyanosis and the oximeter read 85% saturation. What is the diagnosis **(Fig. 1)**?

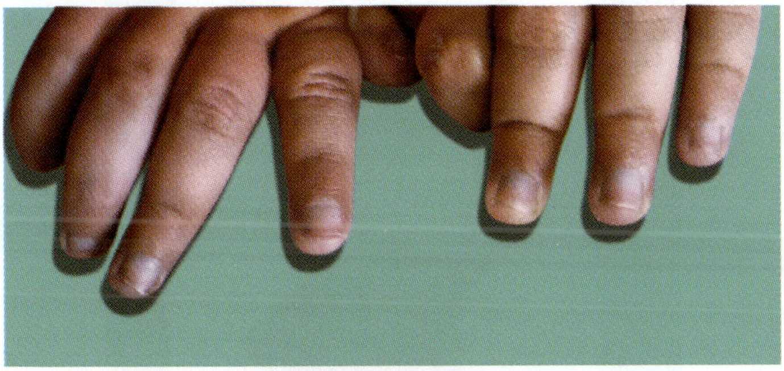

Fig. 1: Cyanosis.

Pause and think before you click the answer:

Answer: The diagnosis could be any form of cyanotic congenital heart disease, but then why the question? Please notice that the child has no clubbing. If you have significant cyanosis and no clubbing, wonder that it could be methemoglobinemia! Further, the oximeter in methemoglobinemia would show 85% due to the instruments inability to distinguish oxy and meth hemoglobin (HB). Since methemoglobin absorbs both the spectra of light used to identify deoxy and oxyhemoglobin, the saturation is unreliable and is low despite normal or high pO_2. If the methemoglobin levels are 30% or more, the saturation plateaus at 85%. Further, on exposure to air, the blood-containing methemoglobin remains chocolate brown, as seen in this case also, whereas the cyanotic CHD child's blood would turn pink (upper frame CHD-shown for comparison) **(Fig. 2)**.

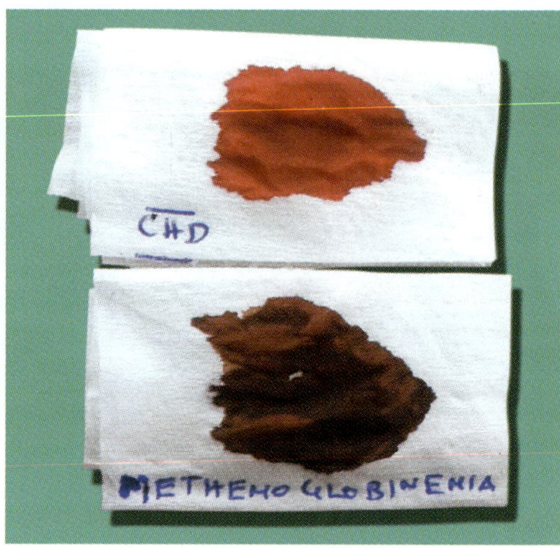

Fig. 2: Blood on exposure to air.

Learning point: Methemoglobinemia does not cause clubbing.

Sidelights: Acquired methemoglobinemia may result from oxidant drugs or chemicals like benzocaine, lignocaine, dapsone, nitroglycerine, nitric oxide, or using water from the wells (in neonates—remember?). In infants <6 months, methemoglobinemia might occur from gastroenteritis and sepsis due to large number of nitrite reducing bacteria and ease of oxidation of fetal hemoglobin.

Methylene blue therapy should not be given to glucose-6-phosphate dehydrogenase deficiency (G6PD) deficient patients as it would cause severe hemolysis.

Very severe methemoglobinemia might require hemodialysis and exchange transfusion and hyperbaric oxygen [extracorporeal membrane oxygenation (ECMO)].

- Argyria—blue to gray skin and mucous membrane might result from chronic silver exposure can be confused with cyanosis (actually should not be confused).
- Red fingertips (tuft erythema) may occur from slight reduction in arterial oxygen saturation as in small or intermittent right-to-left shunts. It is not commonly recognized.

Sidelights:

1. **Which saturation is more reliable—obtained from the blood gas or measured by an oximeter?**
2. **What is the difference between oximeter and co-oximeter?**

Answers: The blood gas estimates the saturation from the pO_2, whereas the oximeter measures it.

- Co-oximetry devices use at least four wavelengths of light to measure not only oxy- and deoxyhemoglobin, but also other forms of Hb (e.g., CO-Hb and Met-Hb).

CASE

42

Echo in a Patient with Palpitation

"Only connect..."

—EM Forster

A 20-year-old had an echo done for the complaints of atypical chest pain and palpitations. The echo is shown in **Video 1**.

Video 1

His ECG during an episode of palpitations is shown in **Figure 1**.

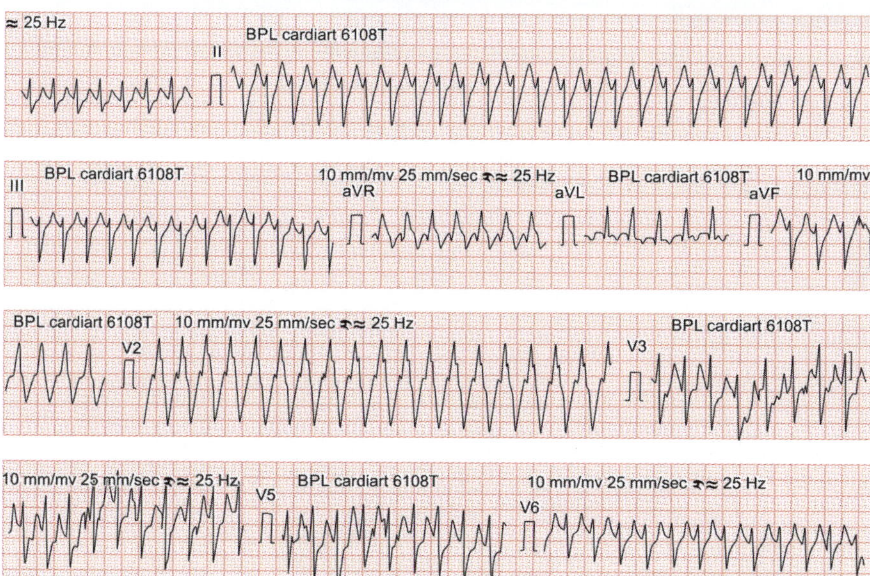

Fig. 1: ECG during palpitation.

What does the echo show?

Pause and think before you click the answer:

Answer: The echo shows a peculiar regional wall motion (RWM) abnormality that is reminiscent of left bundle branch block (LBBB), but it is even more so. Thus the echo is suspicious of a LBBB or a bypass tract causing this RWM abnormality. The resting ECG is shown below **(Fig. 2)**. The ECG during symptoms shows a wide QRS tachycardia (Fig. 1). The MRI subsequently also shows cardiomyopathy with prominent noncompactions of the ventricular muscles **(Fig. 3)**. Incidentally, the bypass tracts are also seen in noncompaction cardiomyopathy, though echo in bypass tracts with no other abnormality may also show such RWM abnormalities. Our understanding of noncompaction has evolved further (noncompaction might be seen in many muscle disease and not a specific entity as previously considered).

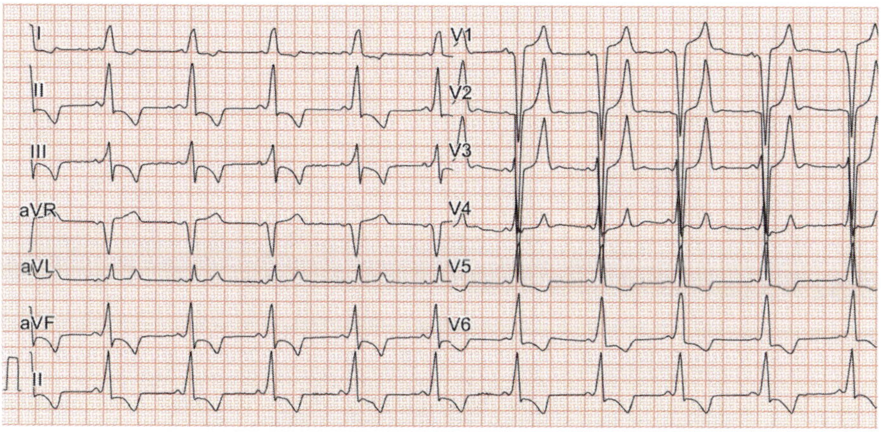

Fig. 2: ECG.

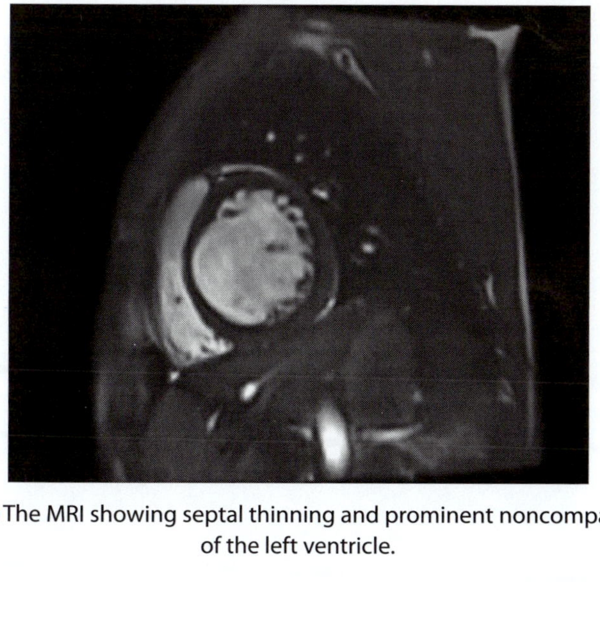

Fig. 3: The MRI showing septal thinning and prominent noncompaction of the left ventricle.

Learning points: Bypass tracts can cause significant RWM abnormality. Ablation of bypass tract in people without any arrhythmia might improve ventricular function in some cases.

Sidelights:

1. **Can a Mahaim fiber show RWM abnormality as shown here?**
2. **Basal septal thinning is suspicious of what diseases?**
3. **What causes septal beaking and septal bounce?**

Answer: Mahaim fibers with decremental antegrade (only) conduction most often have only subtle ECG abnormalities in sinus rhythm. Thus they are unlikely to have such RWM abnormality. During tachycardia, LBBB morphology is seen and that might show a RWM abnormality.

- Basal septal thinning is suggestive of cardiac sarcoidosis or ischemic heart disease with myocardial infarction, trauma (and rarely seen in giant cell myocarditis).
- Septal bounce is seen in constrictive pericarditis (CCP) (case 16) and is due to differential filling velocity of right versus left ventricle in the rapid filling phase. It is seen in every beat and is not due to respiratory changes as often mistakenly believed. Septal beaking is seen during pre-ejection period in patients with LBBB due to ventricular dyssynchrony.

CASE

43

Arm Weakness in an Adolescent

"It takes something more than intelligence to act intelligently."

—Fyodor Dostoyevsky

A 15-year-old boy presented with weakness, pain, and difficulty in lifting objects with left arm for the past 2 weeks. There was no history of fever, trauma, or repeated use of the left arm. On examination, all the pulses in the left arm were very feeble. All other pulses were normal and systemic examination was unremarkable. A chest X-ray was considered unremarkable **(Fig. 1)**.

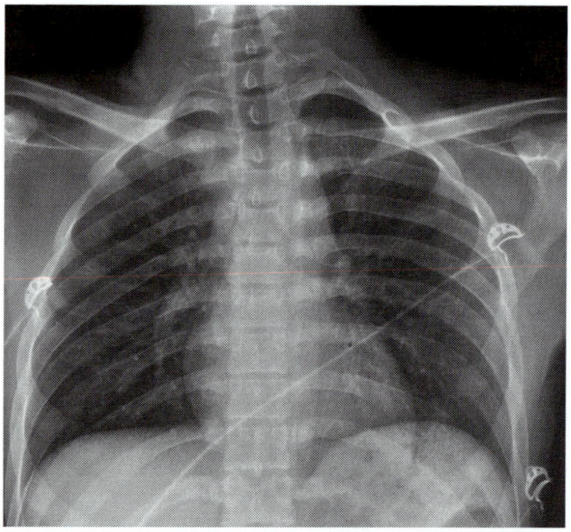

Fig. 1: Chest X-ray.

A CT angiogram showed subclavian artery occluded **(Fig. 2)**. The patient was started on heparin and subsequently on warfarin with which he reported some improvement. There was no family history of similar illness or other thrombophilia. How should he be investigated?

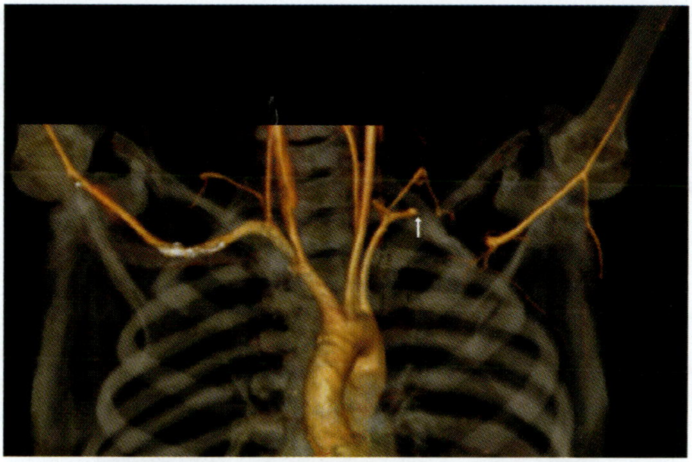

Fig. 2: CT angiography showing subclavian occlusion.

Pause and think before you click the answer:

Answer: The CT angiography picture is typical of an arterial thoracic outlet syndrome (aTOS). The chest X-ray also shows slightly abnormal first rib course on the left side. Although it is not a cervical rib, it is important to consider thoracic outlet obstruction in this case. The bony thorax in the CT **(Fig. 3)** showed indeed it is an arterial thoracic outlet due to pseudoarthrosis of the first rib with the second rib (black arrow).

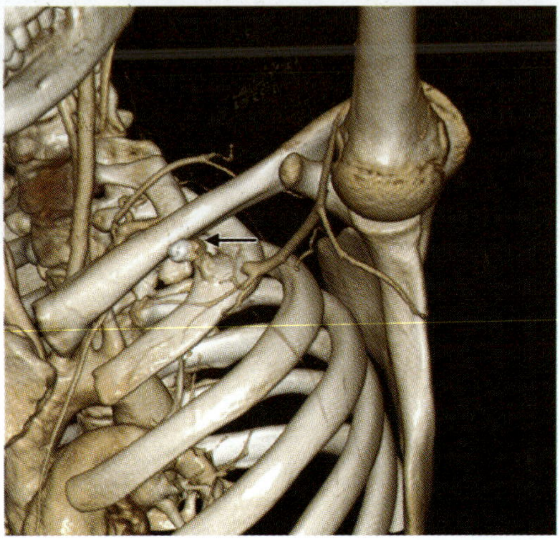

Fig. 3: Thoracic CT showing pseudoarthrosis of the first rib (arrow).

Thoracic outlet syndrome may present with many different neurovascular symptoms. aTOS is rare but important cause of limb ischemia. The subclavian artery compression may result in arterial aneurysm and thrombosis and that may cause acute limb ischemia. Rarely, the thrombosis may propagate retrogradely causing stroke. Cervical rib may be a pointer to the diagnosis, although many other bony abnormalities might also cause aTOS. Cervical rib, anomalous first rib (as in this case), or anomalous muscular bands compressing the vascular bundle must be suspected in a young patient with aTOS. An eminently treatable lesion, aTOS should be considered in the appropriate settings.

(*Source:* Kothari SS, Champaneri B, Panchal N. Arterial thoracic outlet syndrome in an adolescent. Ann Pediatr Cardiol. 2023;16(4):301-2.)

Learning points: Arterial thoracic outlet syndrome is rare, but important cause of limb ischemia, and might occur from causes other than cervical rib also.

Left subclavian artery is the most common artery involved in Takayasu aortoarteritis as well.

Sidelights: Neurological thoracic outlet syndrome may present to the cardiologist with chest pain radiating to left arm and other nonspecific symptoms such as dizziness. An appreciation of this fact might avoid many unnecessary investigations and clarify the diagnosis in many patients. The neurologic TOS might occur due to fibrous bands or anomalous muscles compressing the brachial plexus. Unilateral Raynaud's phenomenon may occur from neurologic TOS due to compression of lower brachial plexus that carry sympathetic fibers.

CASE

44

A Blalock–Taussig Shunt

"The most beautiful experience we can have is the mysterious."

—Albert Einstein

A 4-year-old child had tetralogy of Fallot (TOF) with severe cyanosis. He underwent a Blalock–Taussig (BT) shunt. In the postoperative period, a loud continuous murmur was heard. The chest X-ray showed some cardiomegaly as expected after a BT shunt. However, his symptom did not improve much. When presented to us, the angiogram is shown in **Video 1**.

Video 1

What do you think is the problem?

Pause and think before you click the answer:

Answer: The shunt was mistakenly done to the pulmonary vein as shown in the angiogram. That resulted in the presence of a loud murmur but no significant change in symptoms. The patient underwent a corrective surgery of TOF with takedown of the shunt.

Facts are stranger than fiction!

- A patient of operated TOF presented to OPD with the object shown below. He coughed this foreign body one morning without any other major complaints. Can you identify the specimen **(Fig. 1)**?

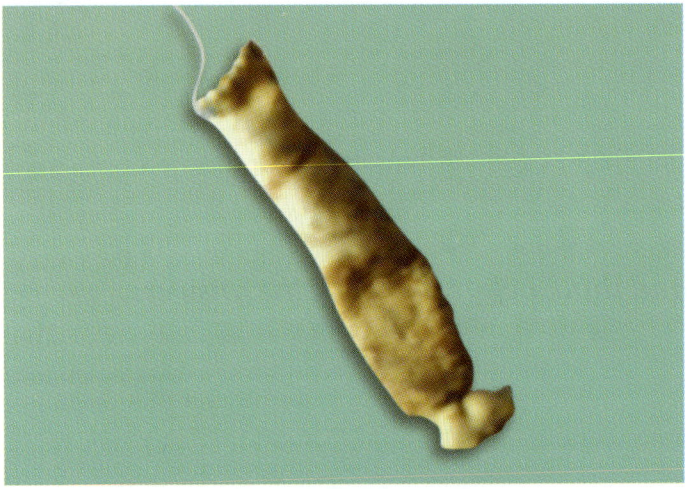

Fig. 1: Patient coughed up this foreign body.

Yes, it is a BT shunt that was done a decade earlier. The computed tomography (CT) of the patient did not pick up any other abnormality like cavity or consolidation **(Figs. 2A and B)**.

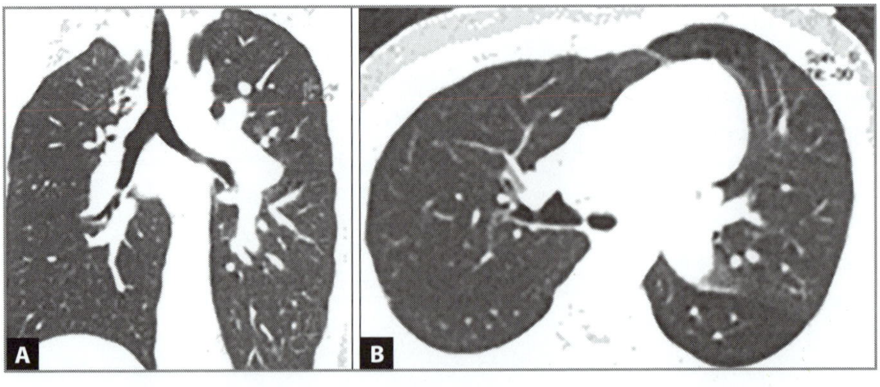

Figs. 2A and B: Thoracic CT did not show any relevant significant abnormality.

A small air-filled diverticulum was seen in the virtual bronchoscopic reformatted images from where the shunt exited **(Figs. 3A and B)**.!!

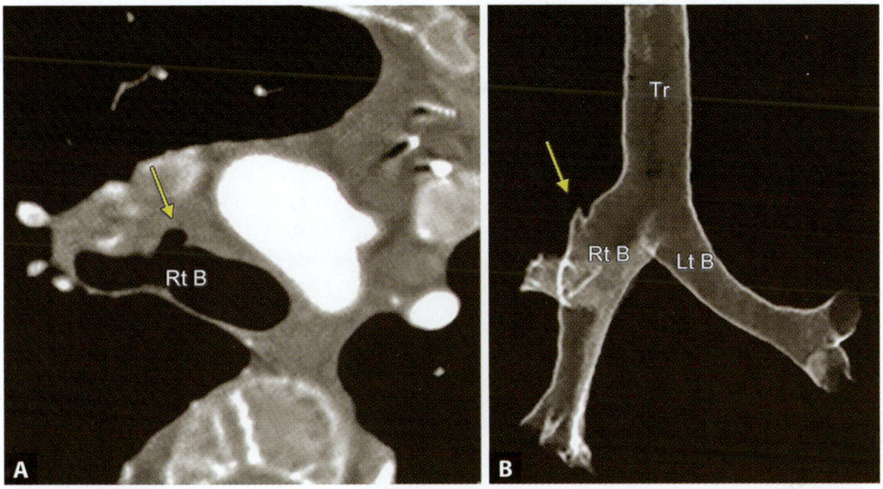

Figs. 3A and B: (A) Oblique axial view of CTA. (B) Virtual bronchoscopy reformat image, anterior oblique projection view, showing a small air-filled diverticular out pouching (yellow arrow) arising from the anterosuperior wall of the right main bronchus (Rt B) and is directed anteriorly and superiorly. (Lt B: left main bronchus; Tr: trachea)

(*Source:* Kothari SS, Murugan MK, Chowdhury UK. Spontaneous expectoration of a Blalock-Taussig shunt a decade after operation. Ann Pediatr Cardiol. 2015;8(1):47-9.)

Learning points: Facts may be stranger than fiction.

Sidelights: Placing a coronary bypass on a coronary vein, ligating the pulmonary artery (PA) instead of patent ductus arteriosus (PDA), closing the atrial septal defect (ASD) by stitching the eustachian valve by the surgeons have all been rarely reported, just as connecting atrial leads to the ventricle or placing the pacing lead in the left ventricle by the cardiologists!

While we are talking of a BT shunt, see this X-ray of a child few months after a BT shunt. How to account for this shadow **(Fig. 4)**?

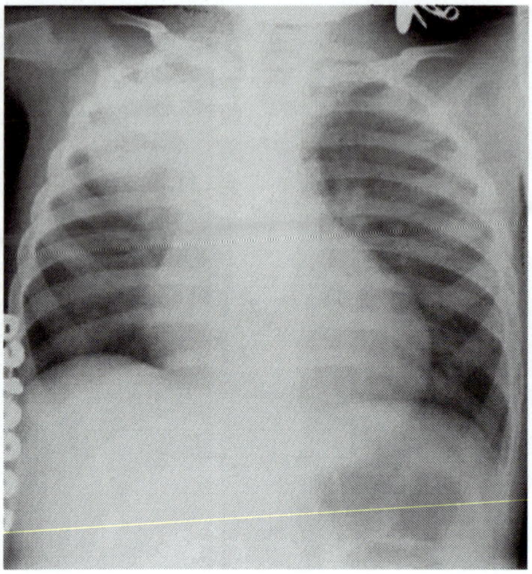

Fig. 4: Chest X-ray months after a BT shunt.

The picture is typical of a seroma that rarely happens after a BT shunt when the serum leaks through the graft. It is rarely seen now a days. The shadow may persist, but is harmless. Since the fluid is rich in proteins, it does not get infected.

CASE

45

Atypical Chest Pain

"The world is full of obvious things which nobody by any chance ever observes."

—Arthur Conan Doyle

An adult male had atypical chest discomfort and no other symptoms. There was no history of fever, chest trauma, or weight loss. His echocardiogram is shown in **Video 1**.

Video 1

Another similar case is shown **Video 2**.

Video 2

What possibilities would you consider?

Pause and think before you click the answer:

Answer: These are the examples of cardiac hydatidosis. An intramyocardial hydatid causing a disruption of the ventricular muscle is seen in the first case. A less malignant form intraseptal hydatid is seen in the second case. Two examples of pericardial hydatid cysts are shown below **(Figs. 1 and 2)**.

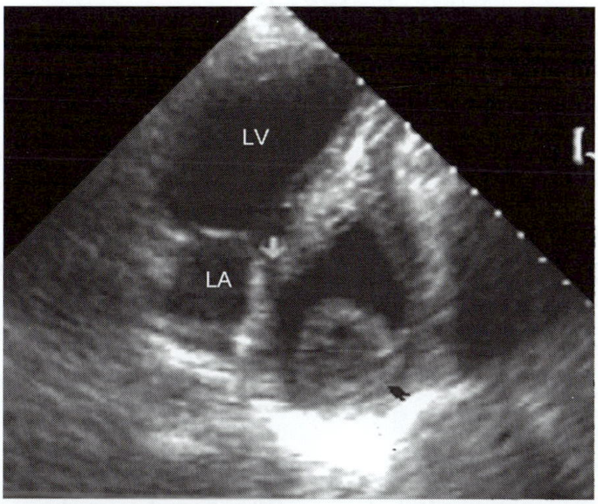

Fig. 1: Echo showing a pericardial hydatid cyst. (LA: left atrium; LV: left ventricle)

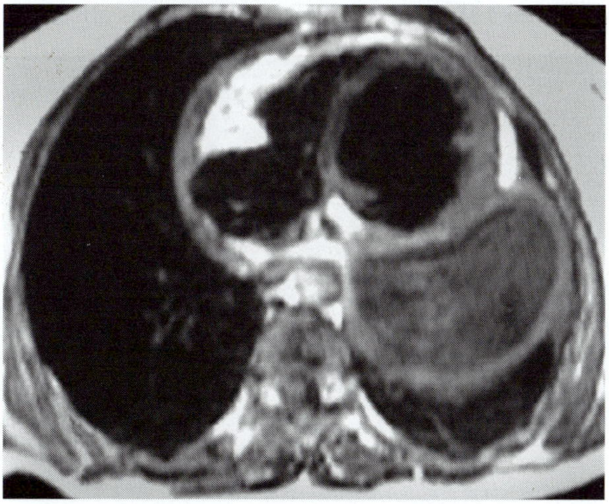

Fig. 2: Cardiac CT showing a pericardial hydatid cyst.

(*Source:* Gulati G, Kothari SS, Sharma S, Bisoi AK. Pericardial hydatid cyst. Indian Heart J 2002;54:437-38.)

A differential diagnosis of the same disease is shown in **Video 3**, though poor record, still it shows an extreme case of a different disease.

Video 3

This one illustrates a very rare example of sinus of Valsalva rupture in the interventricular septum that might mimic a septal hydatid cyst.! (See case 5 as well).

Learning points: Cardiac hydatid cysts can have varying echo pictures and should be kept in mind for the diagnosis of any unusual mass in a context.

Sidelights: Myocardial abscesses may also be either cystic or solid on echo.

See below a rare myocardial abscess **(Fig. 3**, red arrow) in a patient with IE caused by *Stenotrophomonas maltophilia*—a bacteria known to cause myocardial abscesses! The abscess might be missed unless one is familiar with it. See the **Video 4** showing vegetations as well as abscess.

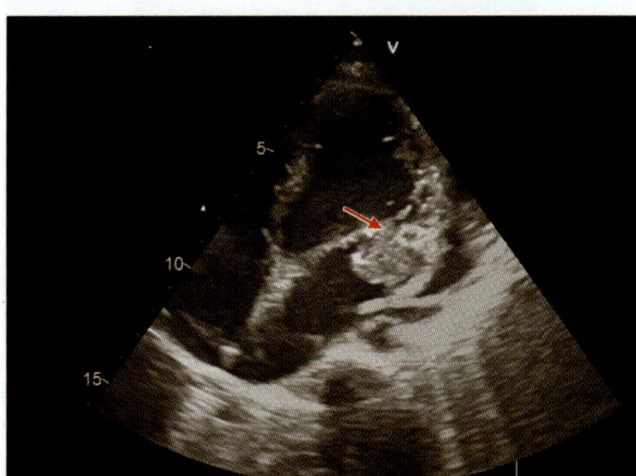

Fig. 3: Myocardial abscess (red arrow).

Video 4

Can you identify what is the cystic structure in the echo below **(Figs. 4A and B)**?

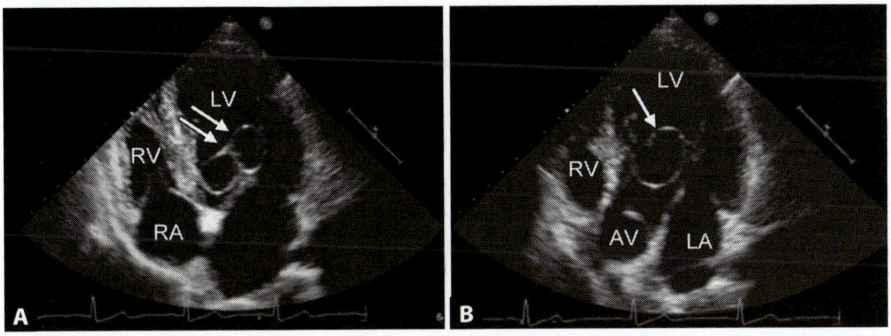

Figs. 4A and B: Echo showing unusual structure (arrow). (AV: aortic valve; LA: left atrium; LV: left ventricle; RA: right atrium; RV: right ventricle)

It is a blood cyst on mitral valve. Blood filled cysts are very rare, not well understood endothelial lined cysts filled with blood. These are more commonly seen in infants and disappear on their own. But it could be acquired and seen at any age; and could cause embolism, valve dysfunction or outflow obstruction (as in this case) and might require surgical removal. The resected specimen is shown below **(Fig. 5)**.

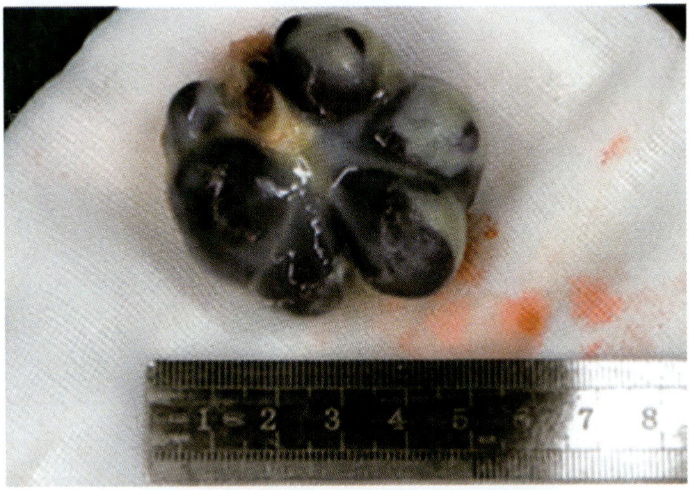

Fig. 5: Resected blood cyst from the same patient.

(*Source:* Ma X, Zeng X, Wu Y, Dong L, Yu Z, Li J, et al. Mitral valve blood cyst occlusion of the aortic valve leading to syncope: detection by transthoracic and contrast echocardiography. J Int Med Res. 2019;47(8):3487-90.)

CASE

46

A Patent Ductus Arteriosus?

"Men live the brink of mysteries and harmonies into which yet they never enter, and with their hands on the door-latch they die outside."

—Ralph Waldo Emerson

A 9-year-old boy was brought with the diagnosis of a patent ductus arteriosus (PDA) for further management. He had a continuous murmur at the second right intercostal space and cardiomegaly. His angiogram is shown in **Video 1**.

Video 1

Can you identify the problem?

Pause and think before you click the answer:

Answer: The aortogram shows only two arteries arising from aorta, right common carotid, and right subclavian (see frame by frame—the silhouette of brachiocephalic seen which is not filled from aorta, but from the collaterals in the brain). The patient has a right aortic arch therefore the left brachiocephalic trunk. In the later frames, the left brachiocephalic and a PDA are seen filling the pulmonary arteries. In fact, his clinical examination showed that the left hand less well developed than right and the pulses on left subclavian and left carotids were weaker **(Fig. 1)**.

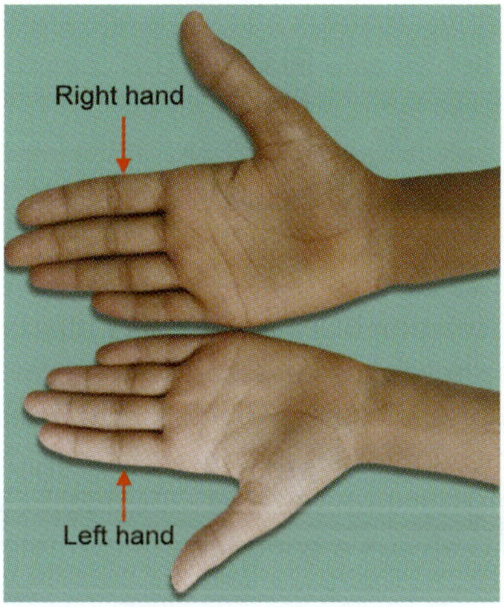

Fig. 1: Left hand is less well developed.

A CT clarified the anatomy **(Figs. 2A and B)**.

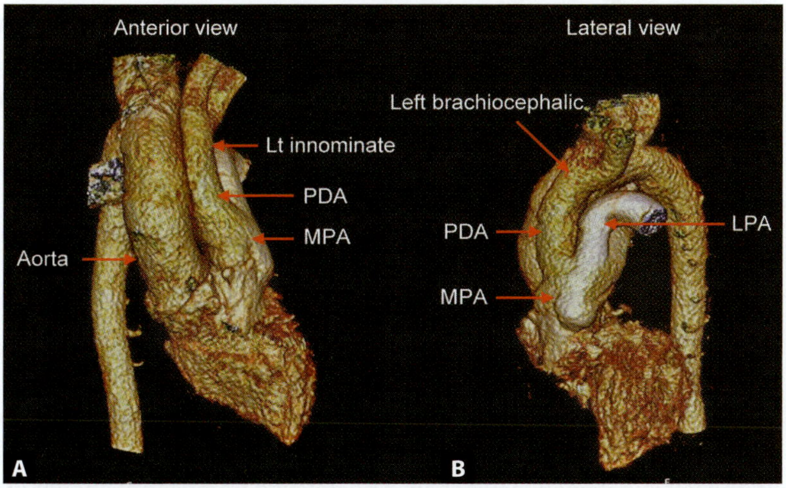

Figs. 2A and B: Reconstructed anterior and lateral view of the CT aortogram showing the left innominate artery from the pulmonary artery. (LPA: left pulmonary artery; MPA: main pulmonary artery; PDA: patent ductus arteriosus)

He underwent successful reimplantation of brachiocephalic to aorta surgically.

(*Source:* Dubey G, Gupta SK, Kothari SS. Isolated left brachiocephalic artery with the right aortic arch: A rare differential of large patent ductus arteriosus. Ann Pediatr Cardiol. 2017;10(1):78-81.)

Of additional interest was the fact that the right coronary artery also arose from the pulmonary artery as shown in the selective coronary injection **(Video 2)**.

Video 2

Learning points: An isolation of a carotid artery may be confused with PDA. Physical examination showing weak carotid or subclavian pulse can prevent a misdiagnosis or a disaster. Isolated subclavian arteries are more commonly known in tetralogy of Fallot (TOF) patients, and not identifying it and going for a Blalock-Taussig (BT) shunt on that side may be disastrous. Palpating pulse of the patients is always a good idea in cardiology, and elsewhere in medicine in general.

Sidelights: Reimplanting a carotid in such cases leads to cerebral edema after 24 hours. Such reperfusion cerebral injury is prevented by clonidine pretreatment! Such cerebral hyperperfusion is also seen after carotid stenting occasionally, especially if patient had chronic severe carotid stenosis and hypertension after stenting.

See the Video 3—can you spot the problem?

Video 3

This is to reemphasize the isolation of arch arteries. In this case of TOF patient, the left subclavian is not seen. The delayed frames (not shown in the angiography) showed left subclavian connected to pulmonary artery.

CASE

47

PAH sans PAH

"No problem can withstand the assault of sustained thinking."

—Voltaire

An 22-year-old patient was referred for complaints of exertional breathlessness and fatigue. Shown below is the echo of the patient that shows severe tricuspid regurgitation (TR) and right ventricular dysfunction. The patient was managed as a case pulmonary hypertension elsewhere for sometime but he did not improve. The pulmonary arteries were not well visualized because of chest deformity **(Videos 1 and 2)**.

Video 1 **Video 2**

Subsequent tests showed no pulmonary stenosis (PS) or pulmonary arterial hypertension (PAH). What could be the reason for this severe TR and right ventricular dysfunction in the absence of pulmonary hypertension or PS?

Pause and think before you click the answer:

Answer: The patient X-ray is shown below for your perusal if you have not got the answer **(Fig. 1)**.

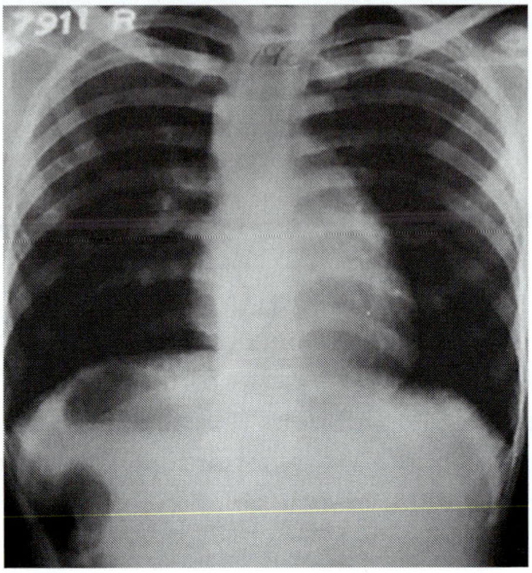

Fig. 1: Chest X-ray.

Now do you know the answer?

Click again if you don't.

As you can see, the patient had situs inversus and corrected transposition with levocardia. The right ventricle was systemic ventricle that was connected to the aorta and not to the pulmonary artery (PA). His PA pressure on cardiac catheterization was normal. Once the possibility of situs inversus is brought in, rest all fall in place (this patient was actually diagnosed as PAH and right ventricle failure by a cardiologist!)

Learning points: In adults with corrected transposition (who typically have mesocardia and sometimes poor echogenicity because of that), misdiagnosis might occur unless situs, atrioventricular (AV) and ventricular-arterial (VA) relations are systematically analyzed.

Sidelights:

1. **How do we get the His bundle tracings in corrected transposition patients?**
2. **What is the longevity of a patient with corrected transposition and no associated heart defects?**

Answers: The conduction system in corrected transposition of the great arteries (CTGA) patient and situs solitus is displaced. The heart block is much less common in CTGA patients with situs inversus. Due to displaced His bundle, the His bundle signal may be obtained from aorta. There may be two AV nodes as well.

- Patients with CTGA and no associated defects have lived up to 90 years! But it is rare to have CTGA and no associated defects. Patients of CTGA and mild PS or an ASD (with small-to-moderate shunt) should not be treated for these lesions as these lesions prevent septal displacement and possibly delay the tricuspid regurgitation so frequently seen in CTGA adults (Just as the PA band in these patients is recommended to treat TR). So remember no PVBD for mild to moderate PS, or ASD device closure for small ASD in CTGA!

CASE

48

Aortic Aneurysm

"The task is not so much to see what no one has seen, but to think what nobody has yet thought, about that which everybody sees."

—Erwin Schrödinger

A 40-year-old lady had complaints of breathlessness and chest discomfort on exertion. The evaluation revealed an aortic aneurysm **(Fig. 1)**. There was no history of hypertension, family history of aortic disease, or clinical findings suggestive of Marfan's syndrome. The face gave away the diagnosis **(Fig. 2)**. Can you point that out?

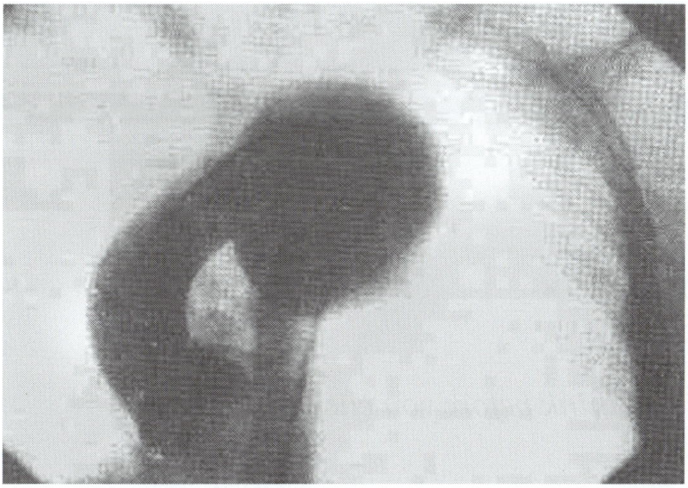

Fig. 1: Arch aneurysm seen on aortogram.

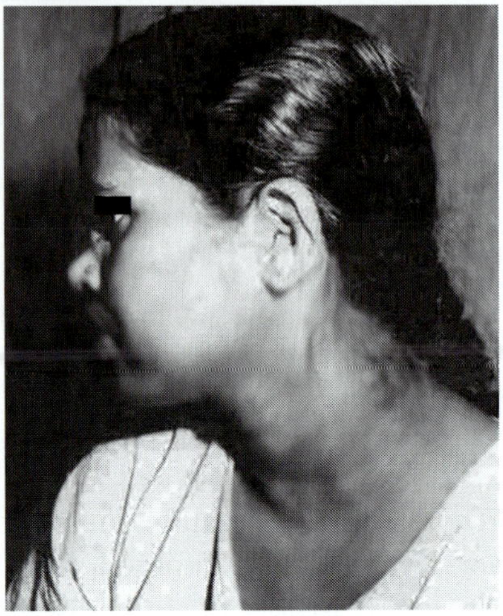

Fig. 2: Photograph of the patient (with permission).

Pause and think before you click the answer:

Answer: The patient had relapsing polychondritis and aortic aneurysm. The face shows the collapse nasal bridge and the ear cartilage. Retrospectively, there was a history of episodes of nose and ear inflammation was obtained that clarified the clinical picture.

- Similarly, in another patient with aortic aneurysm and having features of Marfan syndrome, the oral cavity examination showed the following **(Fig. 3)**:

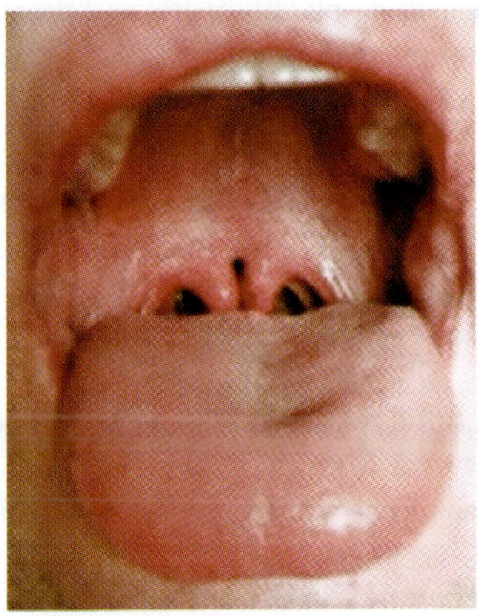

Fig. 3: Another patient with aortic aneurysm, oral cavity (original picture lost; this is from the internet).

What is the diagnosis?

Answer: The bifid uvula in a patient with aortic aneurysm should support the diagnosis of Loeys–Dietz syndrome that involves mutation in TGF-β signaling pathways. The vascular pathology in Loeys–Dietz syndrome is more aggressive than in the Marfan syndrome and hence the distinction might be clinically important. Bifid uvula, though may be seen in normal individuals, or may suggest submucosal cleft.

Learning points: Relapsing polychondritis, a systemic vasculitis affecting many organs, is an uncommon cause of aortic aneurysm. There are no specific diagnostic tests for relapsing polychondritis and there may be overlap with other systemic autoimmune disorders.

Sidelights: So often face tells the diagnosis, but we see the monitors instead! Or the history tells the diagnosis but we see only the images.

Shown below is the volume rendered CT image from a 10-year-old girl with a massive aortic aneurysm from the ascending aorta and proximal aortic arch **(Fig. 4)**. The cause of this aneurysm was not clear until the history was obtained.

The patient had fallen flat on a stony surface while running 2 months earlier. The aneurysm is severely compressing the right pulmonary artery. She developed pericardial effusion after the injury and the aneurysm could be mycotic aneurysm from infection extension, but it was traumatic aneurysm at surgery.

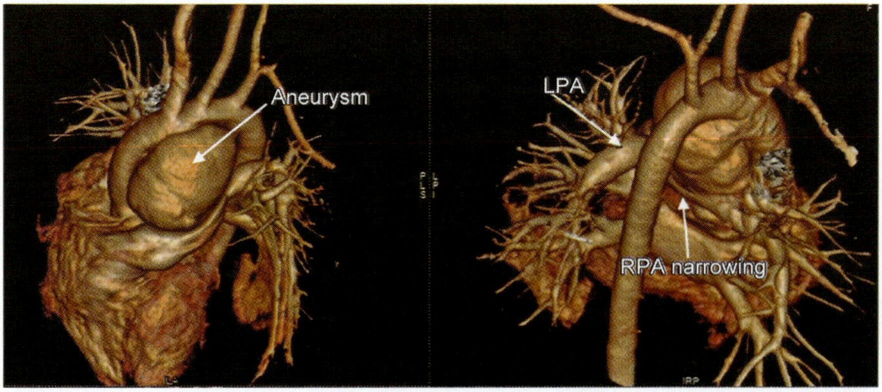

Fig. 4: Massive aortic aneurysm in a 10-year-old girl compressing right pulmonary artery.

CASE

49

Typical Chest Pain

"A fault gets aggravated if it is concealed but fades away if revealed."
—Ganesh Puran

A 50-year-old man presented to emergency at midnight with chest pain. His blood pressure was 170/100 mm Hg. He was not known hypertensive, diabetic, or a smoker. The ECG is shown in **Figure 1**. The troponin level was mildly elevated.

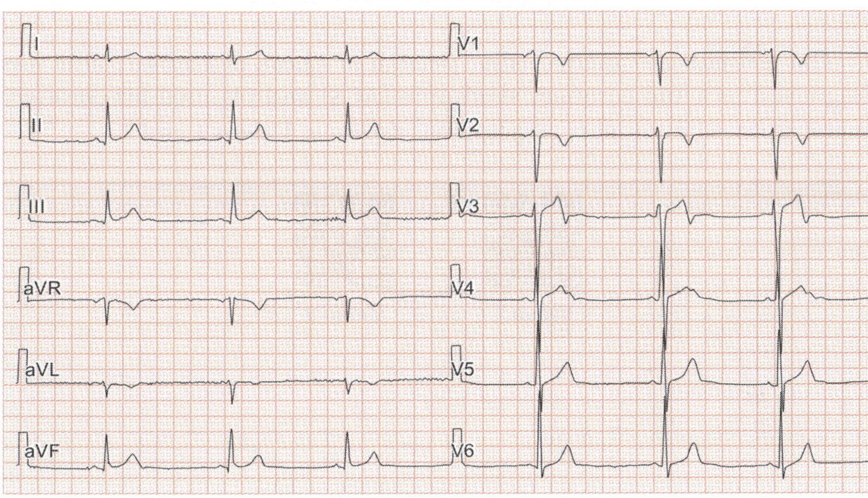

Fig. 1: ECG at presentation.

A repeat ECG when presented to another hospital is shown below **(Fig. 2)**.

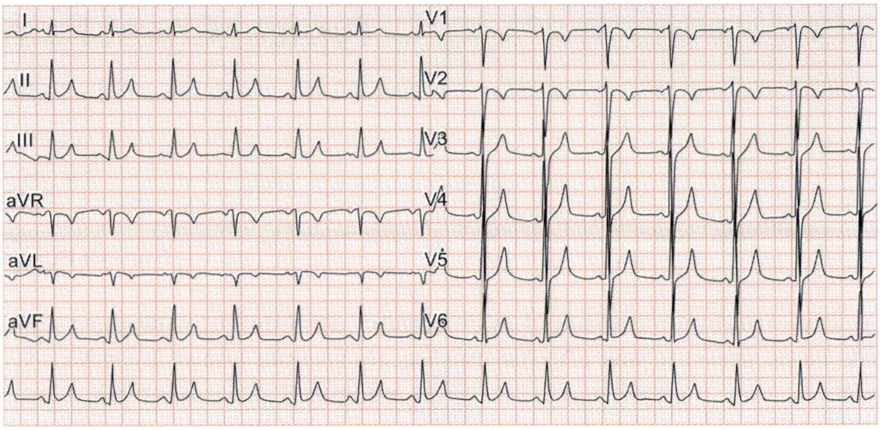

Fig. 2: Repeat ECG after a few hours.

The patient had tachycardia, persistent chest discomfort and was diagnosed as acute coronary syndrome (ACS) and planned for coronary angiography. The coronary angiogram is shown in **Videos 1 and 2**.

Video 1 **Video 2**

The coronaries are nearly normal. The patient collapsed half an hour after the angiography. What is the diagnosis? The angiograms are giving the clue.

Pause and think before you click the answer:

Answer: Look carefully at the angiogram. It shows pericardial effusion. The patient had an aortic dissection. A CT angiography was done after the patient collapsed and was resuscitated **(Fig. 3)**. The coronary angiogram would have worsened it. Retrospectively, lack of ECG changes, weaker femoral pulse as compared to radials, mildly elevated troponins, and pericardial effusion should have alerted to the correct diagnosis. The echo was not done immediately prior to the procedure. Presence of mind could have picked up the effusion seen during the coronary angiogram on fluoroscopy.

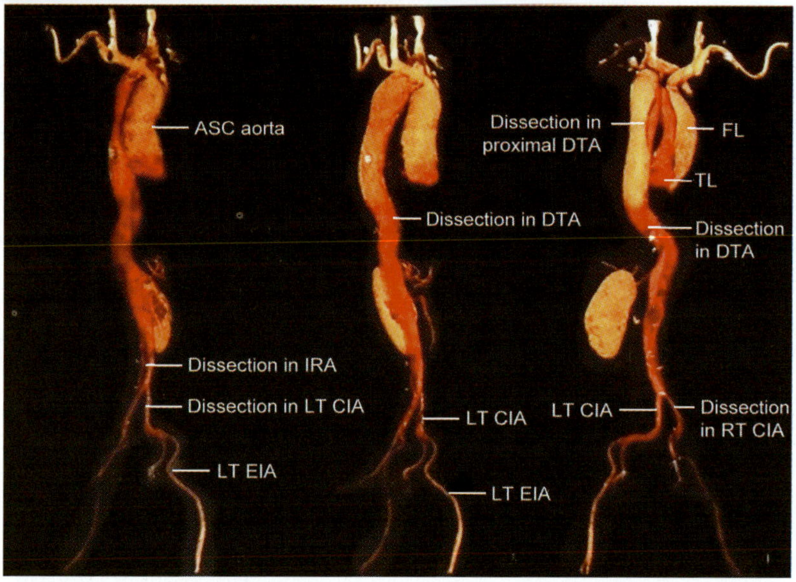

Fig. 3: A reconstructed CT aortogram. (FL: false lumen; LT CIA: left common iliac artery; RT EIA: right external iliac artery; TL: true lumen)

The patient died while being prepared for emergency operation.

Learning points: The fact that aortic dissection might present as acute coronary syndrome is elementary, but it should strike the clinician at the right time.

Sidelights: The dissection when extends distally, it does so to the left iliac 90% of the times. The true lumen is almost always smaller than false lumen. Visceral ischemia occurs in 20–30% of dissection due to compromise of branches in the false lumen. Pleural effusion in aortic dissection patient might be due to aortic rupture and hemothorax, but might also be secondary to inflammatory response and exudative effusion.

CASE

50 Therapeutic Misadventures

"Kindness in words creates confidence. Kindness in thinking creates profoundness. Kindness in giving creates love."

—Lao Tzu

Finally, this series shows some therapeutic misadventures. You might have read about them, but seeing these pictures would possibly reinforce the fact that complications are best PREVENTED. Because, these are obvious, there are no question and answer in the last session.

A. The patient had a neck swelling that was biopsied in some local hospital, the swelling grew rapidly after that **(Fig. 1)**.

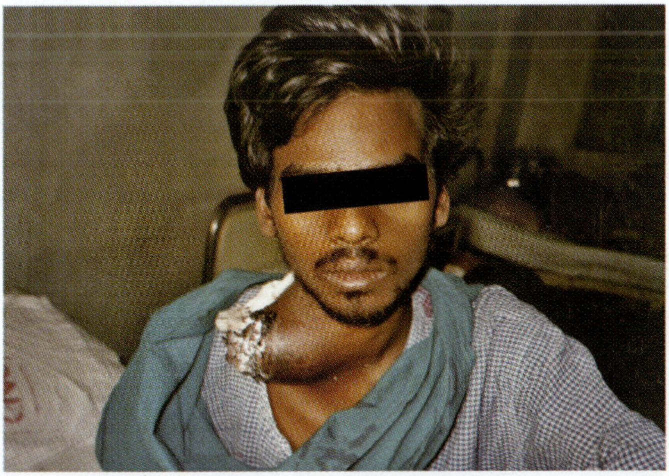

Fig. 1: The neck swelling.

Obviously, it was a carotid aneurysm. The patient was successfully operated.

B. A 20-year-old girl was a known patient with multiple inoperable coronary cameral fistulae. She had chronic hypocalcemia. She presented to emergency service with complaints suggestive of tetany. After some treatment for tetany, she had the facial edema and swelling in the upper half of the body **(Fig. 2)**.

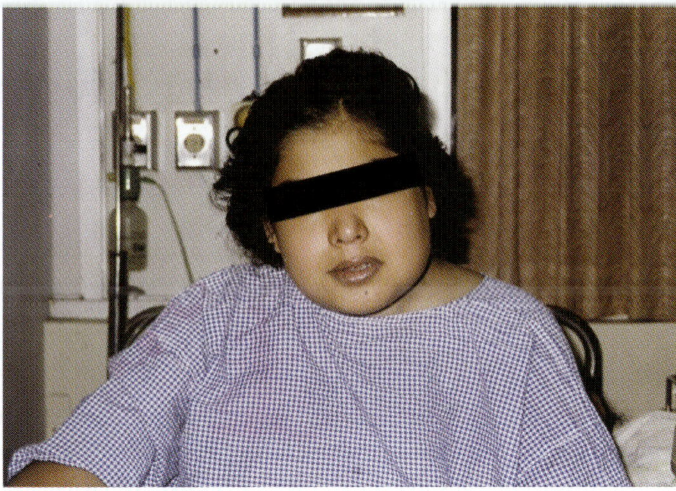

Fig. 2: Facial swelling after some treatment for tetany.

She had received calcium intravenously that caused thrombosis of the veins even up to superior vena cava (SVC). An apparently simple therapy ineptly done can be life threatening. The patient died from unrelenting SVC thrombosis and cerebral edema.

C. A 5-year-old child had congenital heart disease for which a Blalock–Taussig (BT) shunt was done during infancy. A preoperative catheterization prior to corrective surgery was done. Hemostasis was seemingly adequate. After 12 hours, the patient started oozing and had this result **(Fig. 3)**.

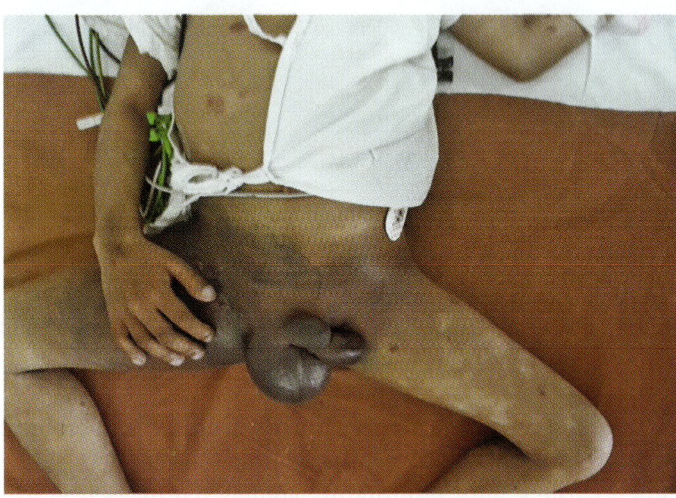

Fig. 3: After an uneventful cardiac catheterization.

The patient had hemophilia that was undiagnosed and caused delayed bleeding. On retrospective review, child had somewhat prolonged bleeding after the BT shunt surgery that was not investigated and considered secondary to platelet dysfunction.

D. A 50-year-old lady in the intensive care unit for acute renal failure, and sepsis requiring ventilatory support and frequent sampling. She had radial artery thrombosis and the gangrene of the fingers. Her ulnar artery was hypoplastic **(Fig. 4)**.

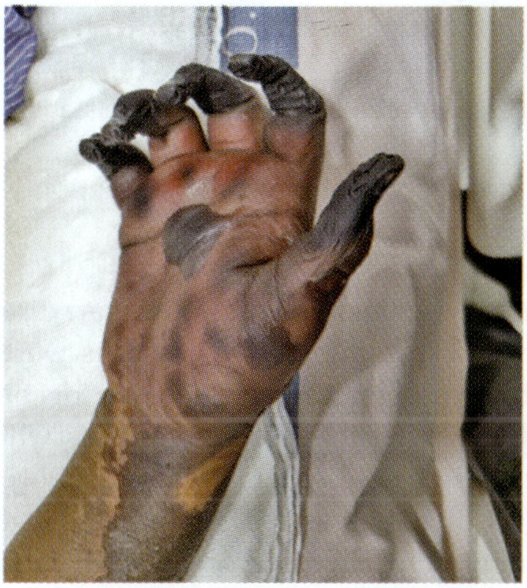

Fig. 4: Gangrene from radial thrombosis and ulnar artery hypoplasia.

E. A 23-year-old patient with coarctation of aorta underwent balloon dilatation of the coarct. The gradients were abolished with the balloon. The pictures before and after are shown in **Figures 5A and B**. Anything more is required? The angiographies are shown pre **(Video 1)** and post **(Videos 2 and 3)**.

Video 1 Video 2 Video 3

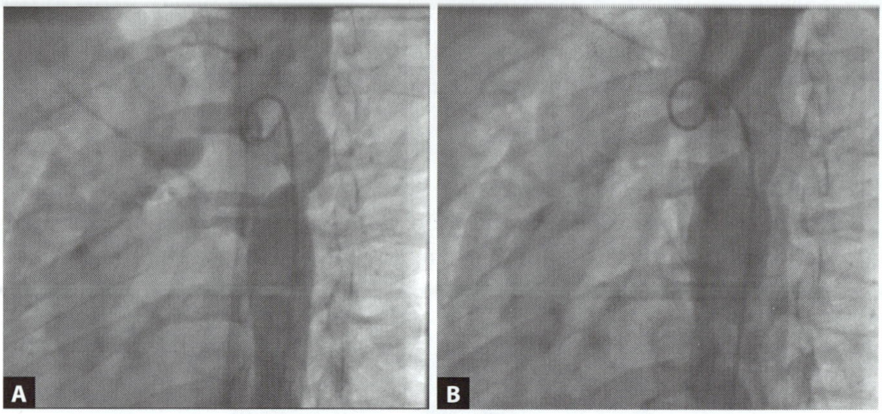

Figs. 5A and B: (A) Before and (B) after balloon dilatation of coarctation.

The patient did not report pain and the dissection was entirely missed. The patient collapsed after few hours.

F. A 10-year-old child with operated cyanotic heart disease presented with hemoptysis. The aortopulmonary collaterals were embolized using Gelfoam since they were small and not suitable for coil embolization. The procedure was done by an experienced radiologist who is well versed with the issue of spinal artery embolization. The child developed quadriplegia after the procedure due to spinal cord infarction **(Fig. 6)**. On retrospective review, no collateral supply to spinal vasculature could be identified. The MRI showed cervical cord infarction **(Fig. 7)**. The child improved slowly over a year with four-fifths power in upper limbs and three-fifths in the lower limbs.

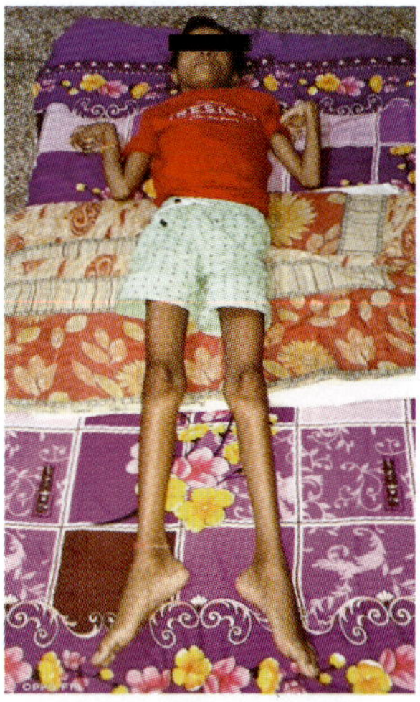

Fig. 6: Quadriplegia after coil embolization for hemoptysis.

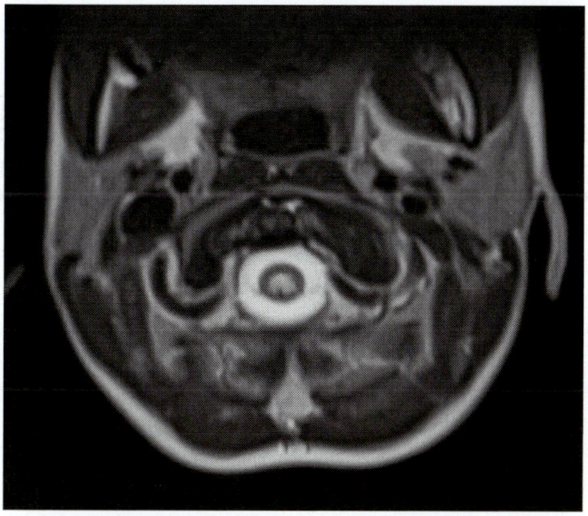

Fig. 7: MRI showing cord infarction.

These rare but striking examples should be remembered as a further resolve to improve clinical evaluation and clinical care in our lifelong quest for learning. But let it not depress you, for these have been extremely rare examples picked up with great difficulties for educational purpose.

With best wishes......,

Endnote

"Life is too short to waste
The critic bite or cynic bark,
Quarrel, or reprimand;
'Twill soon be dark;
Up! mind thine own aim, and
God speed the mark!"

—Ralph Waldo Emerson

Index

Page numbers followed by *b* refer to box, *f* refer to figure, and *t* refer to table.

A

B

C

D

E

Q

R

S